FREE FALL

FREE FALL

by
JoAnn Kelley Smith

Foreword by Dr. Elisabeth Kübler-Ross

JUDSON PRESS, VALLEY FORGE

FREE FALL

Library of Congress Cataloging in Publication Data

Smith, JoAnn Kelley.
 Free Fall.

 Includes bibliographical references.
 1. Breast — Cancer — Personal narratives. 2. Smith,
JoAnn Kelley. I. Title.
 RC280.B8S55 248'.86[B] 75-6690
 ISBN 0-8170-0684-2

Printed in the U.S.A. ⊕

Cover Design and Illustrations,
Agora Inc., Minneapolis, Mn
Art Direction, Joan Radosevich

926.16994
5651

Acknowledgments

. . . to Gene Trumble and other members of the board of trustees of the S. T. McKnight Foundation for their support and encouragement, which have made this book possible and have given my life new meaning.

. . . to Gladys Karhu, who invited me to share my experiences with her students at Mounds-Midway School of Nursing, Saint Paul, Minnesota, and opened the door for a whole new vocation for my life.

. . . to L. M. Conley, executive director of Midway Hospital, and his staff for the conscientious care I have received as a patient.

. . . to Nanci, who transformed the tapes of my addresses into a manuscript for publication.

. . . to my physicians for care beyond their professional oath.

. . . to more than thirty foster sons and daughters, who have given me a reason to live.

. . . to the Agora Community for their unfailing support of our Home of Agape.

. . . to my family, whose love sustains me.

TO:

Mel and Muriel, Ray and Gladys, Jack and Elizabeth, Dick and Barbara, Pat and Alec, Harold and Kathleen, Alice and Ruth, Marcy and Gordon, Lloyd and Lois, Tom and Pat, and John and Carol for their persevering love through a crisis which has dramatically changed Gordon and me.

41962

Foreword

I am sitting next to my Christmas tree which is ready to be taken down. The branches are dry and the candles can no longer be lit because of the hazard of fire. Besides hundreds of Christmas cards there are boxes of manuscripts to be read hopefully before the holidays are over and routine work starts again. My initial reaction should perhaps be "another book on death and dying" — being impressed by the flood of publications in this relatively new field of Thanatology. Then I start to read and read on, and I know that this book *has* to be published and spread, and read by many people. It is not just another book on dying, it is almost a diary of a young woman and mother, wife and Christian, who is willing to share with us her struggle with her faith and her cancer. It points out how little our theology has dealt with death itself but also reminds us of Jesus, the man, who himself passed through the stages of dying carrying his cross.

Somehow the dying Christmas tree next to me — usually a symbol of joy, birth, and gifts — reminds me even more of the shortness and value of life while for a few hours I have the privilege to share the beauty and struggle of life with JoAnn Smith.

What makes this book so real and thus so helpful is the fact that it is filled with humble humanness and honesty. It is written even with a sense of genuine humor — which, unfortunately too many people lack and too many regard as simply being flippant. To face the reality of death requires a sense of humor as well as of personal strength, the courage to question and to tolerate great hostility of pious men and women. FREE FALL is filled with beautiful examples of both: the minister who refused to communicate with her because of her open and honest doubts and questions about life after death; the temptation to be seen as a saint, a super-human being when friends requested her to put in a good word in heaven or "to say hello to my wife."

It is the true story of one person's physical, emotional, and spiritual crisis and experience which lasted for years and is perhaps best summarized in her own words when she writes about the confusion of the dying person: "I am not sure why but I want to accept, and end up rejecting; I want to love but often show hostility; I find peace but am often afraid; I am willing to surrender but more often seek to control; I seek joy and find sadness — and I have faith but live with insecurity."

JoAnn shares with us the loneliness and often dehumanized environment of the hospital where a voice speaks through an intercom

7

and where patients begin to feel like robots. We are beginning to sit with her in a cold hallway waiting and waiting, when the pain becomes unbearable and when she is simply told, "the doctor wants to have this and that" without ever taking her own wishes into consideration. We are beginning to wonder why husbands are not allowed to share the room at night with their dying wives in order to feel some warmth and love when it is so much needed.

FREE FALL is a book of guidance, how to be human and not be ashamed of it: how to understand your moods, fears, and hopes — whether you are the dying patient yourself or a family member or fellow Christian. It is a final plea for you to remain a person and to understand that every human being needs people, needs to be needed, and needs to know that you care. As long as our patients have this kind of genuine love, even a long-term illness will be a growth experience and become an affirmation of our faith. Thank you, JoAnn, for leaving this legacy behind for your husband, your children, and all of us who still have to face this experience.

I have only one regret — namely, that I have not seen these pages until a few weeks after you died. I would have loved to share with you what I know — not what I simply believe — about death itself. Too many have studied dying; too few have done so with death itself. Those of us who have studied what happens to people the moment they die, know that death does not really exist. Only the physical body dies. If you could have listened to those who have died — medically speaking — but made a comeback — and related their experience to us — you would have known that there is no need to fear. It is a peaceful, beautiful experience, a sense of wholeness without fear, pain, or anxiety. I would have liked to tell you that your image of the butterfly suddenly able to move from crawling to a lifting of the wings is the closest to the truth of what already happened to you before I was able to tell you. A "Free Fall" became your image and your expectation — for me it will be a "Free Floating" one day, the direction may be different but since there is no time or space in the beyond — even this will make no difference. Until we meet . . . .

Elisabeth Kübler-Ross
1975

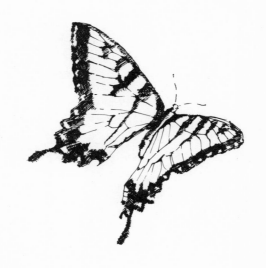

Preface

She was a pretty girl, somewhere in her mid-twenties, and one of the most popular girls on the staff at Midway Hospital, Saint Paul, Minnesota, where I work as Director of Education and Development. A mutual friend had suggested that I talk with her when I had received the diagnosis of JoAnn's terminal condition. "You know she's a widow," he said. "Her husband died of cancer two years ago and she might be able to help you."

I arranged to have lunch with her the next day. As we ate in the hospital cafeteria, she told me she and her husband had married with the full knowledge of his terminal condition. In the freshness of their love, she had encountered anger, bitterness, hostility, and the rejection caused by cancer, a disease which creates the kind of pain and suffering that can alter even the most loving person. Their Christian faith was tried and the hope of their young, romantic relationship went sour under the strain of pain and the haze caused by a variety of medications.

Eighteen months later, a man I had known for over a dozen years asked me to visit him in his office. While we shared a light lunch he asked me how things were going. I sensed his genuine concern and leveled with him. "The emotional ups and downs, the anxiety, the uncertainty, and the inability to continue communicating as we have always done is driving me up the wall," I said. He pressed for details and asked how I was coping with the situation. I told him. He became excited and called his secretary to the office. He asked me to repeat my story for her. I did. Then he said, "Gordon, my wife became seriously ill several months ago and our relationship has deteriorated to such an extent that I almost hate to go home. Our marriage has been happy and our relationship the best but now I can't seem to do anything right and I'm at my wit's end." Somehow we found ourselves sharing our common experiences and searching for ways to live through them.

Knowing that others were facing the same kind of struggle we were facing helped JoAnn and me accept a generous offer by the S.T. McKnight Foundation of Minneapolis to finance the production of a book. We would relate our story, in an open and honest way, for others who might be helped by our experience. FREE FALL is our story. The book is not meant to be a technical analysis of the progress

11

of a disease or a scientific analysis of the body and the physical and emotional reactions to treatment. The best book we have read approaching the subject this way is Stewart Alsop's *Stay of Execution* (Philadelphia: Lippincott, 1973) which we recommend to readers interested in that perspective from a dying patient.

Rather than analysis, our purpose is to affirm the humanness of Christians caught in crisis. We have attempted to relate the ambivalence, contradictions, and emotional conflicts experienced by one who is dying. It was our feeling that more needs to be written about crisis by those who are tasting the bitterness that comes only in the long months of a terminal disease. For this reason, JoAnn and I collaborated to tell her story — our story. It is an account of a Christian family confronting death, as humans experiencing anxiety, hostility, fear, rejection, and hope — the hope that comes from a supportive Christian community where Christ dwells.

Gordon E. Smith

Contents

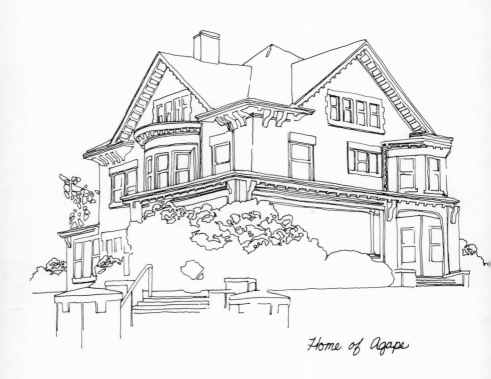

Home of Agape

The fact of the matter
    —just speaking the word
Has an uncomfortable feeling about it somehow.

"He isn't gone; he's just passed away —"
He isn't gone; he's like a bird
Soaring high . . . waiting for us in that

                                    sweet bye and bye.

I never believed I would have to confront a death sentence. Nobody does. And I suppose everyone who does has different feelings about it. But yet I honestly expected it, since my mother died of cancer over twenty years ago at the age of fifty. Cancer's a big thing in our family — my mother, aunts, and several uncles have all gone this way. My mother's began as mine did — in the left breast, then to the right, and to the abdominal cavity.

Still, the verdict came hard. It was terrifying.

John Burns, an internist who had cared for me since 1966 and whom I had grown to love as a person and respect as a professional, was sitting by the side of my bed in Midway Hospital, St. Paul, Minnesota. It was December 16, 1972.

John had been called in as a consultant when I entered Midway on April 22, 1966, with excruciating pain in my chest after having been discharged from the hospital a few days earlier following a hysterectomy. I felt I owed my life to him for he discovered an embolism, a blood clot, which he promptly treated before my condition worsened or I developed a more serious, or even a fatal, embolism.

And on March 26, 1969, he discovered the lump in my left breast and acted quickly to have a surgeon perform a radical mastectomy. Again I felt he saved my life with the early diagnosis and treatment for cancer. In retrospect I realize that as of that date I was never a whole woman again, nor could I ever be.

As a good patient who wanted to live, I came back to John first for three-month checkups, then at six-month intervals as I went into my second year following surgery, then into three years.

                            *   *   *

In 1970, our family made a commitment to begin a group home. We had experienced a degree of success with two foster teenage girls, and our county's welfare department kept asking us to take more.

15

Until April of that year, I did not feel well enough to handle that responsibility. Now we were ready.

Our commitment to do this was strongly rooted in our Christian understanding of mission. The family had grown disillusioned with much of what was happening in the organized church. We found ourselves organizing and raising money to make our church building more adequate and to help "save the blacks in Zaire." While such goals can be important, we felt a strong need for mission as personal involvement in the lives of people who needed what our family had to offer.

I was in middle life and could not see how my energies were really making a difference within the life of my church.

Our family had discussed this problem for many hours and were ready for a positive response when, after Ramsey County Welfare placed two teenagers in our home, we were asked, "Why not consider a group home?" This simply meant the addition of three to four more, which would then form a community in which the young people could help each other work out their problems and reach their personal goals. We had experience in group process, used it in our family, and knew it would work in a group home.

So we sold our four-bedroom home and in November moved into one with nine on the edge of the ghetto, in the inner city of St. Paul.

This decision was supported by a newly organized house church which we joined, the Agora Community. Agora affirms Christian mission as proclaiming the gospel where you are. It provides support, worship, and strong interpersonal relationships to members in their mission.

The word "agora" comes from the Greek New Testament meaning "marketplace." For our family the primary marketplace for sharing the Good News is our home. Without a building, organizational needs for Agora are minimal and so we found the freedom "to do our thing" — providing a Christian home for those who need it. Since then there have been over thirty boys and girls placed in our home. They come from a variety of racial and ethnic backgrounds.

Some have succeeded, some have returned home better able to cope with life, and some have run. One was picked up in New York City and charged with masterminding twenty-seven robberies. She is seventeen. Another, fourteen, has twice run to prostitute in our city and is now locked up. Another, thirteen, did the same thing and gave birth to a baby whose grotesque deformities were probably caused by the mother's extensive use of a variety of hard drugs.

Our group home, which the Agora Community dedicated as the

16

Home of Agape, maintains a normal family atmosphere with Gordon filling the role of breadwinner and a good father figure. I try to be a helpful mother — presenting a positive model of an adult woman. Many of our teenagers have had such bad home experiences that one of the most important contributions we make is that of caring adults, who eventually may become the positive parent models that they often need.

Although our commitment was that of the family's, I viewed our home as the vocational purpose for my life, one which I had sought since our marriage in August of 1949. Here was an opportunity to use whatever gifts I had and the preparation I had in college and seminary within an environment in which I felt the most comfortable — the home.

The name "Home of Agape" was chosen because in Greek *agape* means a love which goes beyond that of brotherhood or of romantic love. I interpreted it to each boy and girl as a "tough love." I would love them whether I liked them or not, approved or disapproved of them. If they ran, if they rejected me, if they deceived me — I would still love them. And we hoped this feeling would prevail in the home and eventually transfer to them. As we saw that happen, the group began to share responsibility for each other.

* * *

On August 6, 1972, going into the fourth year, working toward the five-year anniversary of my first mastectomy when the lucky ones are pronounced "cured," John Burns found a small lump in my other breast, the right one. Although he could not diagnose this accurately without a biopsy, I was certain that again the worst fears I had harbored since my mother's death had come true. Intuitively I knew I had cancer. Only this time I had some firm convictions about how this would be handled.

When the first mastectomy was performed by an excellent surgeon with whom I enjoyed a very warm personal relationship, I was told that the normal surgical procedure was to remove the lump and take a frozen section while I remained on the operating table. Then, if it was malignant, the radical surgery would be performed.

When I asked John how I would know whether or not I had cancer he said, "You'll know — if you wake with a terrible burning sensation on your left side — you will know we had to remove your breast." I remember waking to that terrible pain and Gordon trying to reassure me that all would be all right. "Only one of twelve nodes was affected — they got it early and think you'll be all right," he said.

But for those four years I harbored the deepest of resentment against the medical profession, especially for male doctors. As hard as I've tried, I can't get over the personal feeling that many doctors flippantly hack away at womanhood. I know that the surgeon sees his responsibility to remove all abnormal tissue and does it. But it seems to me this is often done regardless of the emotional consequences to the patient.

I never got over feeling that I was less of a woman because of these surgical procedures. And I believe that I should have been consulted concerning whether or not the breast was to be removed. In our culture this procedure cannot help but do permanent psychological damage to a woman. And the Reach for Recovery Program, at least for me, is not the answer. It seems too superficial and appearance-oriented.

My problems are deeply rooted in who I am as a sexual being. I feel that sexuality has been taken from me. I needed help in learning to accept myself, and I needed preparation for the new life-style which would surely follow such a radical procedure.

So, when the second lump was discovered in August of 1972, and John suggested a biopsy, I was prepared. "Only on condition that it be done as an outpatient," I said. "After the diagnosis, I'll decide what to do." He told me, "That's not the way it's done." I said, "Then no surgeon will cut me again."

Now John is a tough, brilliant Irishman. We share the same national and emotional heritage. No one is going to control either of us. Even if I am a full foot taller than he is, I can't control the way he treats me either professionally or personally. He was in the upper part of his class in medical school and a chief resident during his training. So he's used to winning.

He's not the kind of physician the nurses like to see coming, but he's great for his patients, because he's quick to chew out nurses if they make a mistake. And very few people slap him on the back and say, "Hi there, how are you?" He's not the type.

He was so distressed by my attitude that he left the examining room in anger and returned only after he had regained his composure.

The surgeon who had performed two earlier procedures was a close friend and would have done as I requested, but he was out of the city and unavailable at this time.

So John finally agreed to try to find another who would do it the way I wanted — "but that may be impossible," he said. "You better," I replied. "I'm tired of arranging my life for the convenience of the medical profession. Now they can do it for me!" My hostility was intense, but John and I had an understanding and a deep respect for

18

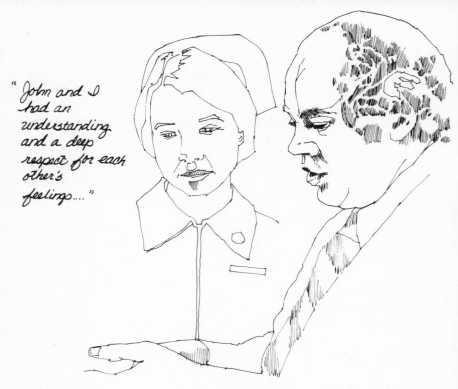

" John and I had an understanding and a deep respect for each other's feelings...."

each other's feelings. He often dealt with me that directly. Now it was my turn — and he understood.

One of the strong convictions I have out of this experience is that a woman should have the right to be brought back into consciousness after a breast biopsy and have several hours, or even days, with her husband, priest, minister, or friend. Then she can determine for herself exactly what she wants to do. She needs emotional and psychological help even if it messes up medical procedure. In my opinion the critical question is not what works best for the doctors and the hospital staff, but what offers the best opportunity for the patient's emotional, as well as physical, recovery.

The next day I reported to the hospital emergency room, and the procedure took place about 10:00 A.M. All that was used to deaden the pain was novocaine. I was awake to talk with the surgeon and to make a usually very competent nurse so nervous that she kept dropping her instruments. The surgeon held up the tiny lump, showed the nurse and then me and said, "It looks benign — a malignant lump is less circumscribed."

I got dressed, went home, and cooked dinner for nine people that night.

But when the lab report came back two days later — his initial

19

reaction proved to be wrong. The lump was malignant — but so low grade that the pathologist said less than six like it had been recorded in the tumor registry of the Mayo Clinic in Rochester, Minnesota. The surgeon, John, and Gordon all tried to reassure me. They said it was not metastatic — had not spread from the other breast. It was a different cancer — low grade, meaning it would not spread rapidly, and the pathologist felt surgery might not be necessary — certainly not radical surgery. But the surgeon said, "The only hope for cure in breast cancer is breast surgery and, as a matter of fact, a case can be made for removing both breasts when cancer is found in either one."

To me, that made some sense. The trauma would be only once. The fear I had experienced for over three years would have been removed. The problem of appearance — balancing a real breast with a prosthetic one — would be removed.

I trusted the surgeon, who proved to be as compassionate as he was competent, and this time felt I shared in the decision. The pain and discomfort of this "simple" mastectomy wasn't as great as the "radical." And, more importantly, the emotional adjustment was much easier, for I shared in the decision — a principle I would stay with through the rest of my days. I would no longer allow others to decide what they would do with my body. They could recommend, advise, but the ultimate decision would be mine — as long as I remained in control of myself.

The next few months turned out to be some of the most frustrating in my life. My anxiety over the future was at a peak. Even our usual two-week vacation at a Northern Minnesota lake cottage with my husband and two daughters didn't help.

My extreme melancholy grew deeper. Nothing seemed to help. John had prescribed antidepressants, stimulants, and a variety of pain medication to control the chronic pain I experienced in my back — diagnosed as mechanical, that is, muscular-skeletal. Even the unusual demands of our six foster teenagers, some of whom were in deep trouble, didn't help. Usually I could lose myself in trying to help them cope with their problems. But even this did not succeed in removing my depression this time.

By November I had my back against the wall — the overwhelming fear of cancer, my physical inability to achieve the goals I had set for myself, and my emotional instability made life unbearable for me — and for the family. I was increasingly slurring my speech and found rational thinking almost impossible.

At this point I did what every woman who endures a mastectomy should do — as an integral part of her treatment. I went to a psychia-

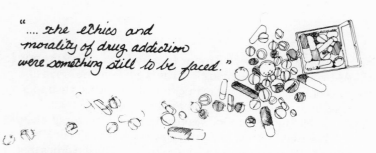

trist. This decision was as hard for me as anyone. I had always been strong-minded, and I had been taught that the Christian faith provided us with answers for every life situation. For me to take this step, I had reasoned, was to deny the relevance of my faith.

By discussing my problems with those who shared my Christian perspective, I had believed that I could get the help I needed. When that failed, I talked with a minister friend who was a professional counselor. Then came several conversations with the hospital chaplain; these helped me gain insight into who I was and what I was experiencing. But I failed to find handles that I needed in order to cope with life as I now found it. I just couldn't get it together.

Gordon finally convinced me that only a psychiatrist could help — if anyone could — for he believed my emotional health was directly related to what was happening to me physically and only someone who understands the relationship between the body and the emotions could help.

It was early in December, 1972, when I finally agreed to have psychiatric help.

I went to a Christian psychiatrist — not necessarily by choice — it just happened that way. He was a man of simple faith — the faith of one who believed that Christ was his Savior, and beyond that he was unwilling to go. Theology, for him, simply messed up his faith. I could respect that, but felt he was copping out and told him so. I also had some problems believing anyone who had not suffered the loss of his sexuality, as I felt I had, could help me.

But Jim did help me. He put me at ease the minute we met. He is a man in his mid-forties, a mod dresser who seems to be at ease in any situation. His office is tastefully furnished and is equipped with the stereotype psychiatrist couch and lounge chair — only he lay on the couch and I sat in the chair.

He is a realist who never let me escape my fear of dying and who affirmed me as a person experiencing the realities of life and death although they were bearing down on me with greater intensity than on many others.

During the first of what was to be a series of psychotherapy sessions,

21

most of which were in my hospital room, he asked me, "What are you taking?" As I enumerated the medicines, he went to a bookshelf and took down a volume describing the drugs and their effects. He underlined each section and asked me to read them.

I remember thinking, "My God, I must be ready to be put away someplace." He asked, "How can I help you — when I can't deal with the real JoAnn?" My personality had been so altered by the drugs that he could not help me deal with my problems.

The use of drugs is something that I have always had difficulty accepting. Many of the foster boys and girls we have taken into our home had used "speed," LSD, or marijuana, had sniffed glue, or used a variety of other drugs or a combination of several. One day I was called to the junior high where one of our thirteen-year-old foster daughters was hallucinating so badly she was completely out of control.

Another night the police brought home one of our fourteen-year-olds who claimed that she had been raped. Wild-eyed and screaming, she shouted, "They're coming to get me again!" The police calmly said, "Pour some coffee down her, and she may change her story." Several times we took girls to the hospital emergency room to have their stomachs pumped because they had overdosed.

I had seen their personalities change within the space of a few short hours from glum introverts to hyperactive extroverts unable to sleep or to sit still. Several times I sat with one of the girls while she came down from a bad trip, and I wondered why anyone would want to do that to herself. Could they be so unhappy with themselves that they needed *that* kind of escape?

Now I was told that in my own way my personality had been altered — through acceptable medications prescribed by licensed physicians. The nature of the drugs and the motivation for taking them were different, but the result was the same. This was a problem I was to deal with many times in the months that followed. And the ethics and morality of the evolution towards drug addiction were something still to be faced.

I left Jim's office that first time with a real sense of hope. That very day, Saturday, I would take no more medication. I would see him one week later, and with a clear mind we could begin to confront the anxieties that were making my life unbearable.

By Sunday I was experiencing some pain but not enough to cause any great alarm. But the next morning I couldn't get out of bed. The pain in my back was excruciating, and my joints ached like a ninety-year-old woman who had suffered arthritis for thirty years. I called

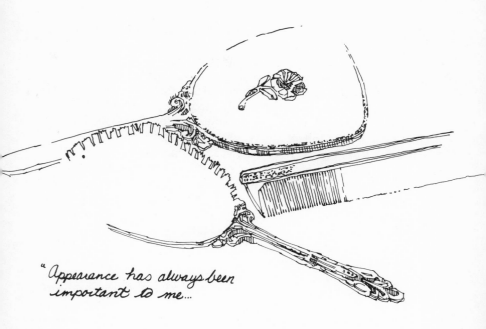

"Appearance has always been important to me..."

Gordon at the office and pleaded for him to get me into the hospital as soon as he could.

As I look back on it now, the pain in my joints was probably caused by withdrawal symptoms.

It was December 12, 1972, when I was admitted for severe back pain by the orthopedic surgeon who three years earlier had performed a laminectomy on my back to repair a ruptured disc. Not only was the pain in my back a cause for concern, but the steady loss of weight also created some problems for which John Burns was consulted.

I had a certain sense of pride in my weight loss. Since August I had deliberately set out to take off some of the fat that I had accumulated in recent years. I was determined to be as attractive as I could — probably overcompensating for the second mastectomy, which I believe made me an ugly creature. I had great difficulty looking at my scars in a mirror, and I never undressed in front of Gordon as my embarrassment and shame were so great.

Appearance has always been important to me, and my family often accused me of being too vain. Vanity is a sin many of us share — but for me it had consumed a great deal of emotional energy since grade-school days when at nearly six feet tall I towered over my peers. My mother taught me to turn my height into an asset rather than a liability. I learned to walk tall, with back erect, to dress well, and to use cosmetics to the best advantage.

The diet was working. I was achieving my goal of a slimmer, neater appearance, but my weight loss now seemed uncontrollable.

John's first examination after I was in a hospital bed indicated that I was in trouble. Flat on my back, weighing thirty pounds less than the last time I had seen him in his office, I could see anxiety all over his face when he was able to feel a mass where my liver is. He said he was ordering a scan. Again I had that awful feeling of terror — that belief that the worst fears I had grown to expect would, in fact, come true.

The liver scan took place late that afternoon in the hospital's X-ray department. There was a sense of urgency about John's orders and the way in which the X-ray techs initiated this procedure. He had to have an immediate verification of his worst fears.

Most of the X-ray personnel had gone for the day except the two girls who operated the scanner, a device which records abnormalities in organs through reaction to nuclear medication injected into the body. I was the only patient left in a normally busy X-ray department. That impressed me with the seriousness of my situation.

My anxiety was so great that I wasn't the least interested in professional ethics or procedure, so I asked the girls, "What does it say?" And they replied, very unconvincingly, "A radiologist will have to read it."

By coincidence, or destiny — whatever your philosophical persuasion — a good friend was right there waiting to walk me back to my room. We had not been as close in recent years as we were when we moved to St. Paul twelve years ago. Both of our families were large and demanding, leaving less time to develop a relationship that at one time had been so meaningful. And we no longer belonged to the same church.

But she had gotten wind of my situation and hurried to be with me. I was so happy to see her — and it was as though we had never been separated. We were on the same wave length and picked up our relationship   where it had left off. Funny how that works with some people.

She took the wheel chair and rolled me back to my room. She wasn't sure what to say — just, "How did it happen?" I said, "I don't know — it just did." And then I said, "Barbara, this is it, I'm sure this is it."

She is, and always has been, extremely healthy, with the vigor of a trim, energetic, and successful mother of six. She asked, "Why does it always have to be you?" The satisfaction of having a close friend with whom I could identify in that crisis moment sustained me for many hours to come.

It seemed to me that within the five minutes that it took to get me back to my room, everyone in the hospital had changed positions in relation with me. I was totally different.

Gordon was home getting dinner for the family, and I had a desperate feeling of loneliness, like being alone on an abandoned ship. I felt no one wanted to enter my room.

I would visualize the nurses drawing straws to see who would enter the only room in the hospital with a "Beware of Patient" sign put there by the executive director, one of my closest personal friends. It was meant to be a joke, but was too prophetic now to be funny.

I needed someone sensitive to what I was feeling — to say or do something — like plump my pillow, give me a pill, or in some way use the skills with which she was trained.

But nobody came. I was just there.

I knew the nurses were all busy.

But in that moment all that mattered to me was me.

I needed someone who would be there with me. I didn't need somebody to tell me what was happening. I didn't need somebody to give me sympathy. But I did need another human who would just be there, and, if nothing else, simply hold my hand until Gordon could get back to my room.

* * *

And now it was December 16, 1972, and John was sitting beside my bed. That conversation was the most traumatic I've ever had, and it stands out in my memory so that I can remember virtually every word.

Tears were freely running down his face. They rolled down his cheeks and off the end of his nose — like a little boy who can't admit to emotion so just lets the tears flow unchecked. He told me that the scan revealed a liver studded with cancer tumors.

Then he told me, "We're in the fourth quarter of the game, and there is no way we can win. You are not going to get better, and there is little we can do for you. I want you to have one more surgical procedure," he said. "I want your ovaries removed to stop the supply of estrogen, which promotes the tumor's growth, and I want a biopsy of the liver so that we can study the histology and the activity of the tumor. This will give us a surer sense of direction in planning treatment."

I tried to relieve the pressure of the personal sense of guilt I thought John was feeling and said, "You've always done your best — you are

25

not responsible — it's just the way things are."

I believe John saved my life three times. Now he was very broken over the fact that he was unable to save my life a fourth time. More important than his extremely fine competence is the fact that he is my friend. I remember that after the second mastectomy, he expressed how unfair it seemed to have my body so defiled.

John is a man of faith. He recognizes the limits of medicine. But he felt, and still feels, that he failed me because he didn't have enough knowledge to save my life. I can't express how much that means to me — to have someone care so much. We cried together as he relayed the bad news.

In order to function in a doctor-patient relationship from this point on, we made some ground rules so that we could cope emotionally with the situation. Dearest of all to me was his confession that in his fifteen years of practice, I was the first patient he really loved that would die. But he said he had now lost his medical objectivity in his caring. He means a great deal to me, and I will ever be grateful for his openness and honesty.

Then I asked him to make a covenant with me: that he would always tell me the truth, that he would not allow me to suffer, and that he would not use heroic methods to keep me alive. He promised, "You will be able to die with a feeling of dignity."

We cannot choose how we are born. But to exercise responsible freedom as a person, we ought to be able to exercise choice in how we die. We ought to be given the freedom to die in dignity rather than exist without it.

Then he asked me, "When you get there — please put a good word in for me." He continued, "If I am a good father, a good doctor, and a good person, please ask God to make a place for me." He was the first of many who have laid that responsibility upon me, mostly all Roman Catholics, who seem to have their afterlife theology worked out much more clearly than do we Protestants. This was a revelation I was to learn in the months that followed.

Because of our close personal relationship and his confessed inability to be objective in a patient-doctor relationship, and because I now would begin chemotherapy, he said he was turning my case over to his partner, Wayne Thalhuber, an oncologist who specializes in the treatment of cancer patients.

After making a thorough study of the histology of the tumor and my body's chemical makeup, Wayne would direct my therapy.

That experience with John was beautiful — and heartbreaking. When he left, I called Gordon, whose office is on the fourth floor.

Gordon is on the hospital's staff and is responsible for fund raising, public relations, and the administration of the hospital's educational programs. I was crying when I told him, "John was here and wants to do a liver biopsy." All Gordon could say was, "I'll be right down."

It seemed like hours. But I discovered later that he had frantically searched the halls of the hospital looking for John and finally found him coming out of the coronary care unit just below my room. He looked at Gordon and said, "I'm not prepared to talk," and Gordon said, "Neither am I, but you must tell me what's going on."

So, standing in the corner, the two men talked. John told Gordon what he had related to me and suggested that Wayne be on the case to administer chemotherapy after surgery. Gordon said, "I don't want to think about that — I can't even talk about that, or cope with that — yet. Let's take one thing at a time." I discovered later that Gordon was opposed to chemotherapy because of the ever-present danger of severe side effects. In a later conversation, Wayne, whose interest in cancer therapy through the use of chemicals had been honed into a fine skill since medical school, convinced him it was our only viable option.

When Gordon came into my room, I discovered that with every devastating experience there are singularly beautiful ones.

Gordon and I have always been extremely open and free. We have tried to be so in accepting others regardless of their shape, form, mode of dress, beliefs, or style of life. And in our own relationship we have been open. But I have been married to him twenty-five years and had never seen him cry.

Now, as we talked, he wept openly. And that demonstrated to me how much he would miss me. I hadn't thought about that very much and it really moved me. It was a very tender moment.

And we talked about how we had always done what we wanted to do when we wanted to do it. We operate on the philosophy of doing today what we had planned for tomorrow. The thought had never occurred, "We must wait until we can afford to go or until the kids are grown." We have enjoyed life together — especially traveling together as a family. We felt we had done the best we could in raising our

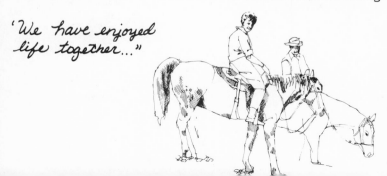

"We have enjoyed life together..."

children and in sharing our lives with those who needed it, the basic commitment of our married lives.

There would be no regrets.

> Life is moving in slow motion at high speed!
> Every gesture, thought and feeling are action packed!
> The days have been good as reality has been recognized
> With friends coming one by one,
> But the nights are long and restless
>   with my mind running rampant
>   over all my feelings, treasured thoughts, precious
>   possessions — treasuring each one.
> How can people hold life so cheap — whole days just wasted —
> It becomes priceless when there is just a little left.
> One feels gluttonous — wishing to clutch
>   at more than one's share
> But one has no right to someone else's precious piece —
> Each must have only one gift of life.

Then Gordon reviewed our theological position, which we had frequently discussed, namely, that "the rain falls on the just and on the unjust." We do not expect God's special intervention for us. We live now as we always have — by the natural law of cause and effect. It is a part of the human condition. If you are stricken with a fatal disease, you will die. It's that simple — and that terrible. Faith in God provides the grace to endure.

And from this stance we started the long ordeal of thoughtful reality.

It's a strange feeling to know that death is now a present reality — time may not be long — and to be told, as John told me, that many will now treat me like a leper because they fear the presence of death which I represent.

No longer will people look at me without having their own mortality called into question. And most people want to avoid that at all costs.

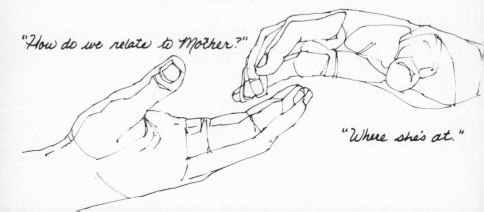

"How do we relate to Mother?"

"Where she's at."

That night Gordon took Paula and Gail out for supper and gently told them that their mother was not going to get better. Paula was seventeen, ready to graduate from high school and Gail was fifteen. Neither girl asked any questions — but Paula understood and, in the effervescence that is found only in teenagers, tried to make the evening pleasant for her sister.

The next day was Saturday and that afternoon Gordon arranged a family conference in the apartment of our nineteen-year-old son, Brian, and his wife, Sally. He simply stated the facts as they were.

It was an emotional encounter. Gail burst into tears asking, "Why didn't you tell me?" Her reaction was simply the proof that we hear only what we wish. Sally's reaction was tinged with the bitterness many feel in similar circumstances, and she probably expressed what Brian was really experiencing in his guts. "If that's the God you believe in, I want no part of him," she said. Paula and Brian raised the practical questions of time. Brian asked, "How do we relate to Mother?" And Gordon replied, "Where she's at." And then they discussed the implications of that.

It has been my feeling that this experience has been hardest on Brian, for I don't believe he has the faith stance to accept what is happening. For him, it doesn't seem fair for his mother, who believes in God, his justice and love, to suffer through the anxiety of four years of serious illness, uncertainty, and the slow process of an incurable disease. Even to affirm a world governed by cause and effect fails to satisfy him.

And for him afterlife is out. On one occasion I said to him, "If you find no need to believe in an afterlife — fine. Then the relationship that you've had with me here is all there is. And if we have failed, then that's very sad." He believes human relationships are circular and when death comes the circle is complete. It is over forever.

This concept is valid for many, and I must admit it has crossed my mind many times. I can accept his stance and often wonder, "What's wrong with believing that this has been enough?"

"That which we are lives on in others," our Jewish friends believe. For them, that gives an eternal quality to the meaning of a family. But it doesn't go far enough for me.

Gordon developed a statement of our faith that night, which he reviewed with me the following morning in my hospital room. I agreed with its contents for we had often discussed the basic theological implications of this kind of situation. Twenty-two years earlier, Gordon preached his senior sermon in seminary and dealt with this very issue.

The statement read:

The meaning of life —
  —the priority of your family
  —the reality of God
  —the supportive love of friends
  —the eternal quality of our existence
have all become the focal point of discussion in the Gordon Smith home.

And now we know that nothing else really matters.

Because we have learned that JoAnn has cancer of the liver and her time with us is limited. She has so much to say to so many people and her energy is limited — so she asked me to write this for us all.

Our family lives with the conviction that God will enable us to be better persons because we can confront the reality of life and death together and together find the meaning there is to be found in this experience. Our life-style has always been open and it will continue to be — that we may learn how to accept the gift of life and how to share with others the quality we have discovered in that gift.

And while this experience offers the truest test of a family's faith and the role of each member — so it does for friends and loved ones who are a part of our supportive community. We are with you as you determine what this experience says to you.

Our God has always been the faithful one who causes "the rain to fall on the just and the unjust." And although we believe that all human destiny is in his hands, we find greater strength in the dependability of his nature. So we have never asked, "Why us?" — but rather "Why not us?" How do we relate to God in this? We ask him to help us find meaning, to give us dignity and inner strength, and to be faithful to our commitments.

When he first learned of this, Brian asked, "How do we relate to Mother?" And in many different ways friends have asked this. My answer to all these questions is, "Where she is." The role of loved ones who really care is to give her the support she needs but to be sensitive to her limited energy and her deep desire to be with those who are closest to her.

A note — a brief telephone call to tell her how you really feel will assure her that those to whom she has meant something really care about her.

We feel that each day — each week — is a gift.

The future is uncertain. But our faith in God and his ultimate purpose is not. And neither is our conviction that in these days we will experience love at a level reached by only a few.

Gordon

The statement was mailed to our friends. We wanted no groups rallying to pray for the unexpected miracle — nor did we want new cures, healers, or quack remedies to cope with or to raise our hopes.

Why should I be spared while three children die of leukemia in the University Hospitals? The miracle came when Wayne found a chemical pack to extend my life beyond the hopes of all the doctors involved in my care.

In my experience with my dying mother I felt that her faith weakened as she sought for a miracle that would restore her health. Well-meaning persons had assured her, as they have me, that if faith is strong enough a miracle will come. I do not believe that attitude helped my father who at that time did not profess a Christian faith. The experience of my mother's crisis didn't help him find a faith. My mother's God failed her — and she was a good woman, he reasoned, so why bother.

Gordon and I would not fall into the easy trap of making demands from God until he gave in. We would accept a miracle if it came as God's gift, but we would not dare plan for it and have the withholding of that gift destroy the possibility of a meaningful faith for our impressionable children. For us, the reality of living through this experience as Christ's people would have a far deeper meaning for our family than would prayers to single us out for the gift of a miracle that might never come.

I do not believe in a capricious God, that he can either heal or take your life depending on the particular situation. This makes a lot of difference as to how a person deals with impending death. Of course, there are some who don't really want to deal with death at all even though it *will* happen to them.

It seems the more pious people are, the more difficult confronting death is because they really don't want to deal with reality. They carefully put any thought of death in some secret box to deal with when it becomes a relevant issue; then they have a hard time because they can't cope with the results. Reality cannot be put off to another day. It's here now!

The ground rules were laid. There would be complete openness — with the family, our friends, and our physicians. And we were all ready, as ready as we could be, for death.

I have often wondered if this is the best stance. It is right, I'm sure — but best, I don't know. Openness can lead to depression, morbidity, and a hostility I never believed could be a part of a Christian life-style.

Stewart Alsop, the respected newsman who died of leukemia in the summer of 1974, recalled the total loss of hope he felt when he was told of his diagnosis. He locked himself in his bathroom and wept. His published story impressed John, who now feels that while the physician should always tell the truth, perhaps it is not necessary to tell all the truth. Instead the patient should be left with some glimmer of hope.

Maybe it would have been better to have left some things unsaid and project some hope that times would be better and normality could come again to our family.

But the die was cast — and readers will have to judge whether this approach would serve the best interest of their own family, if they are confronted with a similar situation.

To have handled this situation any other way would not be consistent with the kind of people we are. Also it is not our style to deal with our crisis without some emotional relief. We have tried never to take ourselves too seriously and therefore our escape valve during my illness has often been humor directed at our own condition, which often embarrasses those around us.

For example, many insurance agents are enthusiastic when we say "yes" to their offer to sell us a policy, but their reaction is uniformly horror when they are told, "JoAnn has terminal cancer — still interested?" In a macabre way, the escape valve is opened and we can joke about it. I often respond to the routine question, "How are you?" by saying, "Sick and dying!" That usually brings the unnerved questioner up short. And for a meeting once I made myself a name tag which read, "JoAnn Smith — a dying person." Because Wayne has been so successful in treating me, I have often referred to him as the physician who took his internship at Lourdes.

So there were several instances in those early days of hospitalization that I can look back at now and find in them a kind of similar sick humor. For example, my dear friend Vince, the orthopedic surgeon who admitted me for back pain, stood at my bedside feeling quite helpless to know what to say now that my terminal disease was diagnosed. But he had an obligation to tell me that the back condition was mechanical and could be corrected by a relatively minor operation — a procedure which now seemed ridiculous in view of the cancer diagnosis. We were both silenced by the ludicrous nature of that situation. It was irony that wasn't funny then, but now in a macabre way it seems to be.

Christmas was coming and I begged very hard to go home if only for a few days. This was considered a very unwise decision by all the physicians, but John relented and said, "Well, let's take a chance." So Gordon brought me home on December 23, and I was there for

32

Christmas Eve and Christmas Day.

On December 27, I was readmitted for surgery to take place the following day.

During my time at home I was very weak and my anticipations were too high. They were unreasonable because I thought this was going to be my last Christmas and therefore would be the greatest that I had ever experienced. Of course, I had very little to put into it so it just didn't turn out as I expected. Gordon's parents came from Omaha to celebrate what might be our last Christmas together since my outlook was not promising and they were now in their mid-seventies. I had some wonderful talks with Grandfather, a minister for fifty years, about death and eternal life. Those conversations offered the best undergirding of my theological stance developed to that point.

On Christmas Day, Ruth and Alice from our religious community visited me. It was Ruth's first Christmas after the death of her mother. I felt that I had also contributed to spoiling their holiday. They assured me that was not so, but rather that they felt so futile — helpless, not knowing what to do or say. "Just being here is the greatest gift of all," I said. Togetherness is a matchless gift. The fact that they cared enough to share Christmas with me was overwhelming. A small share of that Gift of Gifts. Hallelujah!

The round of social occasions during Christmas really turned out to be for me. They weren't planned that way but circumstances made it that way. I became the center of those occasions. However, I had the strange feeling that I was on the outside looking in, a viewer of a provocative film. I began to wonder if this was because my body felt different somehow, or was it because God created in us a state of mind which allows us to prepare for the time of separation yet to be? Do we begin our adjustment to death by growing distant from those we really love?

Sadness of sadness.

A part of the fun of life was departing.

Good-bye, good-bye, forever?

Dream on of Christmas past and present.

Christmas future may never be . . . and I will miss it so.

Will they all miss me too? I'm selfish enough to say — I do hope so.

Merry Christmas!

I felt that the whole Christmas experience was a further extension of my loss of control. Everyone else seemed to be programming and planning my life — physicians, family, friends — as if whatever they could do would alter what was happening or even retard the inevitable. We all seemed to be trying hard to put off that which we feared.

For example, our friends moved up our traditional New Year's Eve party so we could be together once again. Plans were changed so we could all make the date we set — everyone went all out to make it something special. We all tried to be ourselves, but we couldn't. Things were different — they had to be, and I really wasn't a part of it — it really wasn't me.

And my feelings were confirmed by a dear friend who later said that I had a special radiance about me. I became poignantly sad as the evening progressed. I was already experiencing separation from persons I really love.

As Gordon and I left, we both wept as we drove through streets covered with fresh snow. We weren't alone. The group left behind felt the same sad emotion.

Later in that week the experience was duplicated in a visit with other friends. We had had a long-standing dinner invitation and they had done everything they could to make the party the best. Their home was beautifully decorated. The food was great, the guests literate and witty. But I never really felt like a participant, only an observer. When we left, Tom and Pat could no longer role-play. The game was over and we all cried.

Our Christmas interlude was far from what I had told a friend it would be — good food, good music, entertainment, and fun. It couldn't be that because no longer could my body participate in all those things I wanted. It no longer responded as it once did.

Christmas was a dream, and any moment I expected to be awakened — but I wasn't. It was all just as it seemed. Is this what forever means?

Then I found myself wondering, "What if I wake up and it is only a bad dream — what is that dream supposed to say?"

Is that all there is
   these forty and nine
In which to make
   a life enough to be mine?
Cheated, that's what,
Cheated by them all—
Preachers, teachers, mother as well—
Cheated to find that the piece is so small.

Bah, Humbug! It cannot be so—
But you and I know
   in this moment
A pounding blow
   from head to toe . . .
That's it, my friend, that's all . . .
These few passing years before a call
To which we are so ill prepared.
But God, whose fault is it, after all?

"... the whole
Christmas experience
was a further
extension of my
loss of control."

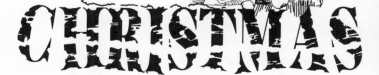

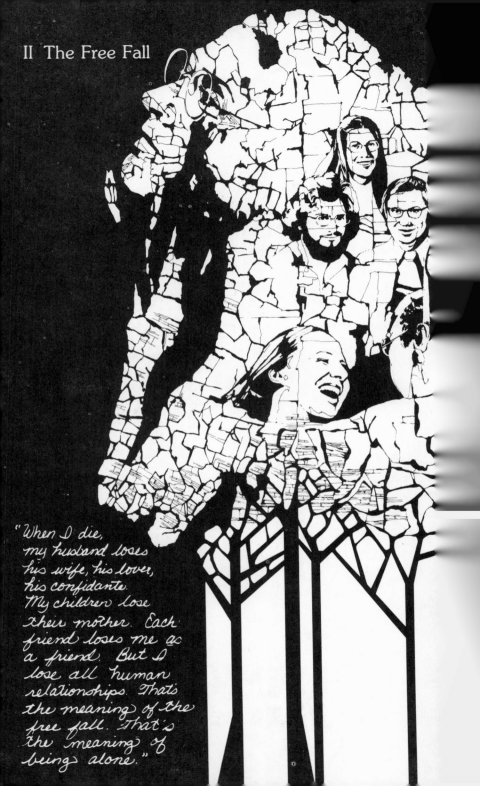

II The Free Fall

"When I die,
my husband loses
his wife, his lover,
his confidante.
My children lose
their mother. Each
friend loses me as
a friend. But I
lose all human
relationships. That's
the meaning of the
free fall. That's
the meaning of
being alone."

In that Christmas interlude we invited our religious community to come to our home because I felt that I would never come back from the hospital after surgery and I wanted to talk with them. The Agora Community to which our family is committed is an experimental house church funded by the Board of the National Ministries of the American Baptist Churches. Our style of worship and study is in small groups, where we share the meaning of our personal faith, often on a one-to-one basis.

I wanted to tell them about my dying and suggest that we talk about it and of what meaning it could have for the whole community. About forty persons came — a community of believers made up of people under the age of fifty with a very high percentage of youth. I sat next to Gail, holding her hand. Later that night she wrote her impressions in her diary. She was touched by the sadness I conveyed as I expressed regrets that I would miss the birth of my first grandchild and would never see my children grow up and mature.

Gordon opened the meeting by saying that I had only thirty minutes and so whatever I had to say I must say in that amount of time because that was all the strength I had to give. Then I would return to my bed while the group had coffee and continued the discussion.

"I want to read our faith statement," he said; "then we can talk from that point." He read the statement emphasizing our hope that we could see this situation through without expecting any special miracle or any unusual deal to be made with God on our behalf. But rather we would try to face it as strong people. As a family, we hoped to move through this experience, learn from it, learn to love each other more, and become able to face death realistically.

After he read the statement, I said that it was terribly important to me that they all know how I felt because of John's comments that "from this point on, JoAnn, you will become a leper."

Before that, I hadn't thought too much about what a leper was even though I had read stories about them in the New Testament. I pondered about what it meant to be one of the despised ones and thought how awful that must have been — totally separated from any social contacts or any loving physical relationships. And I thought of the many modern lepers in our society. We put them where we can't see or relate to them — in high-rise apartments, in ghettos, in institutions, and some in rural settings.

Then I expressed the hope that we could learn something from my experience to give us signposts and help so that we might all gain a sense of security in facing the reality of death. Together this would not be a totally sad experience, but in the end it would be victorious because we all would have learned to celebrate life and its meaning.

There was weeping and a great deal of distress because a number of people really didn't want to believe that I was going to die.

I told them that the best way to describe how I felt is like a parachutist must feel when he leaves the door of an airplane and begins a free fall. I'm falling in very slow motion — ever so gradually leaving planet earth behind and moving into the vast and clear expanse of space.

I have never done this, but according to accounts I have read, the parachute jump comes closest to describing where I am. It is an ecstatic feeling because you are in space — free of time and all restraints.

As long as I have little or no pain, my dying is a freeing experience. Without having to please anyone — released from all inhibitions — I can be totally free to be the person I want to be.

What have I got to lose?

That's a kind of exhilarating feeling.

But at the same time I'm all alone and the farther I fall, the more lonely I feel.

What I asked of the community that night — what I begged of the community that night — was to help me so that my loneliness wouldn't grow until I couldn't bear it. "Don't treat me like a leper," I pled. "Don't separate yourselves from me no matter how ugly I become either in disposition or in appearance. Don't fail to see me because you won't know what to say or because you might cry, or for any other excuse you might discover to escape my presence."

I said, "From this point on I really need you because I feel suspended in space — so lonely here that it almost overwhelms me. Although I'm falling toward a still undefined target below — a center which has meaning, that which Tillich calls the 'ground of all being' — I am alone. But I don't want to be separated from the community which has been my life and support system.

"So when you leave tonight I will probably cry — don't let that be stressful to you because your leaving is a kind of death for me. Each time you leave me, a little of our relationship dies. I give you up a little bit in my free-fall experience. But at the same time I don't want you to give me up. Maybe that's selfish — maybe this is how a dying person expresses his* selfishness — that I want you to stay with me even if I am falling away from you."

I continued, "I want to be close to you and love you. But the aloneness of the free fall takes you away from me. So I need all the

---

* Used in this book, not to denote sex, Heaven forbid, but simply because the familiarity of its use makes for a smoother style and easier reading.

show of love and affection that you can give me even though I can't respond as I once did."

> As each one dear to me
>   Embraces and accepts death's fact—
> I feel myself slipping slowly away
>   Rather like the movement of astronauts
>   on the moon.
>
> I would draw them closer
>   But even as I do, it seems like
>   sand gently falling through my fingers.
>
> How tightly I would hold
>   Yet the grip is ever soft and slipping
>   Away-away-away.
> They hug me, kiss and cry,
>   And the closer they come
>   the greater the sense of awful loneliness
> Engulfs me.
>
> God, you are real only in their
>   embrace, their kiss, their tears.
> Even as I treasure their nearness, they slip away;
>   Is their love slipping, slipping —
> Preparing me for Real Life?

The response of one of my young friends in that group, a sixteen-year-old, was most moving. Because he finds it very difficult to communicate verbally, he wrote me a long letter a few days later.

He said: "I've always been terribly afraid of dying. I think I get this from my father because every time he gets the least pain in his body he just gets panic-stricken. It helped me so much for somebody like you, that I care about, to say, 'Well, you know it's bad but maybe we can work this through and come to some kind of good conclusion.'"

Then he went on to write, "I really appreciated what you said, and I especially like your idea about being in a free fall."

In the months that followed, I found great comfort in developing the concept of the free fall as a means of expressing how I really feel about death, for this concept expresses how the aloneness sets in. There is not a soul to hold your hand or to help you reach your ultimate destination, except for the presence of Jesus, who also traveled this road — to mix my metaphors.

But in our human experience, there is nobody who can help you finally make the break, who can guide you to wherever the fall takes you. You have to do that for yourself. And that is a horrible feeling of aloneness.

When I die, my husband loses his wife, his lover, his confidante. My children lose their mother. Each friend loses me as a friend. But I lose all human relationships. That's the meaning of the free fall. That's the meaning of being alone.

Life is a series of relationships — being together and separating. They are built and broken by our own choosing. So death can be thought of in the same way — as breaking relationships here and establishing new ones somewhere else. But the analogy breaks down. It's not the same. I have not chosen to break off these human relationships that have been so meaningful to me. And my unwanted separation of relationships in death is final — that's the devastating thought. Furthermore, the uncertainty of new ones frightens me.

I've come to believe that my free fall is a kind of preparation for the agony of separation, which is death.

Dr. Elisabeth Kübler-Ross, in her book *On Death and Dying*,[1] implies this too: to have a peaceful death and be able to move from this existence to another, one needs to be freed from all human relationships.

It sort of just happens — or perhaps you do it unconsciously. It occurs in this free-fall concept. The closer I would draw you to me the farther away you move. A little bit — just a little bit at a time.

Therefore, every time I say good-bye, I feel a kind of depression, and a deep sense of sadness as the free fall begins to set in.

This is illustrated by an experience I had when a friend and her husband came from Austin, Minnesota, to see me in March of 1973. Four years earlier she had played a very important role in the recovery from my first cancer surgery. As a physical therapist at Midway Hospital, she had helped to restore the use of my arm. And with her therapy, she restored a good part of my human spirit. She has always been a kind of Savior for my mind and body in crisis. Rita is very dear to me, and she made this trip especially to see me.

Gordon and I had had the joy of seeing her married to a widower with seven children, Jerry Landherr. The two of them came to see me in the hospital soon after the fatal diagnosis. When they prepared to leave my hospital room, all my defenses dissolved as we held each other in the agony of separation. I told her how much I want to stand fast — to be steadfast in the faith which has been mine since childhood, when it was first posited in me by my dear mother.

Rita was a Roman Catholic Sister when I first met her. Although released from her vows to the church, this frail and beautiful woman has a deep faith that enables her to provide spiritual strength to others.

[1] Elisabeth Kübler-Ross, *On Death and Dying* (New York: The Macmillan Company, 1970).

And here she was again when I needed her support and encouragement. I enjoyed being with her so very much, and I will miss her very much. It was very hard to see her go. When the visit was over, I went upstairs, stood at my window, looked out, and with tears in my eyes watched her drive away.

Paula came into the room and asked, "Why are you crying?" And I said, "Because Rita's leaving, and maybe I won't see her again. I must give her up, and every time she leaves I have to give her up a little more. That's really hard because I don't want to do that." I told Paula, "I would like to keep her because I love her. But when she leaves, the free fall begins. You know, a little bit of her goes away from me. It may be a whole lot — I might not see her again. Maybe in this relationship I have taken the whole free-fall experience at once. So the closer I embraced her when I said good-bye to her, and kissed her, the farther away she seemed."

This is the beginning of separation — the free fall.

> How does it feel to be so free
> Yet locked-in ever so tight?
> No song to sing, no flower to see,
> All veiled from earthly sight.
>
> And — the LEAP! — to what, to where?
> O God, my mind has pondered it o'er and
> I find no meaning in the flight
> And fail to assimilate light.
>
> Floating free, destination unknown.
> Believing, but without crystal sight.
> Why do I follow irrational thoughts?
> Maybe because the Bible said so, long ago.
>
> Floating free, hopefully believing
> That all I have been told
>   Will prove real, after all.
> And true reality will be eternity.

Not only does my free fall separate me from others, but there is a sense in which I am also separated from the person I used to be.

To a certain extent I am dead already, for about all I have left are limited creativity and relationships. And I am losing my creativity, and the relationships are slowly becoming tenuous.

As I become more limited, then more of me dies.

It's like jumping out of that plane. When I leave it — the environment I have enjoyed and the relationships I cherish — I begin to die.

41

For me, death is not just the end of breathing or the moment my heart stops beating, but a process. While there is a sense in which all of our bodies are in this process, for me death began in December of 1972 when I was consciously aware that not only was my body disintegrating, but also my person. I can no longer function as I did. It's not there anymore. Those ways are gone. That's death.

When I can't do for other people who have needs and for whom I care deeply, then I realize the process of death has a firm grip on my life.

I don't believe that you earn your salvation by good works, but I think that a God-person, a faith person, isn't really authentic unless he is actively demonstrating his faith. Therefore, I've always cared about people and felt that together, like-minded people could do something to make a corner of the world better. But that desire to be involved with others, and in a cause, is gone because I am no longer able to participate.

If I had been in good health, I would have joined my American Indian friend, Elizabeth Walters Higgins, in working towards greater justice for her people. I would have been involved with the Indian struggle that came into national focus at Wounded Knee in 1973.

But I find myself really having to fight to maintain an interest in any current event. I don't even read the paper; I am not really concerned as I once was with what is happening. I say to myself, "Why get interested — that's dead for me — I can't do anything about it. I can't change it. I can't alter it." Therefore, I begin to rationalize, "Well, as long as I can't do anything about it, why should I show any interest in it?"

That ability to live out an active faith is gone forever; I'll never be able to be involved again.

That's dead for me.

It's lost in my free fall.

42

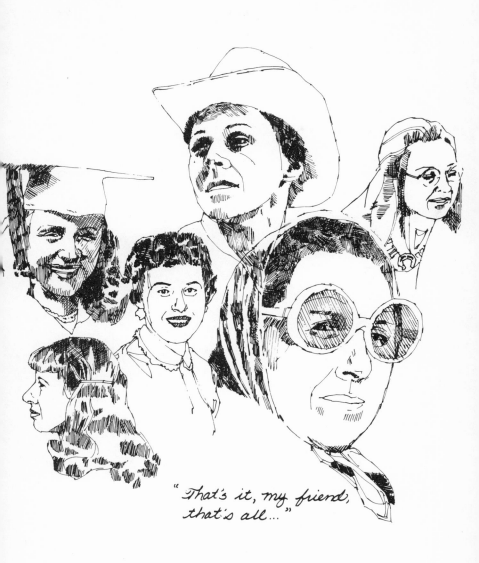

"That's it, my friend,
that's all ...."

III The Struggle for Faith

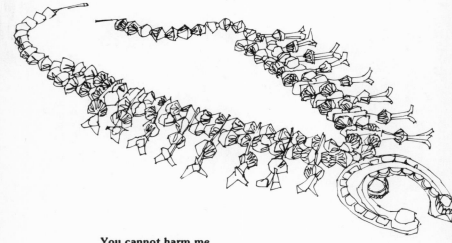

You cannot harm me
You cannot harm
One who has dreamed a dream like mine.

Ancient Indian Poem

"I am filled with the fear that I will not have either the courage or the strength to endure to the end — that I will call out against God and blame others. Then my faith will not, in fact, be real and my life will have been lived in vain."

I confessed this apprehension to my close friend, John Sundquist, who was fulfilling a priestly role in my life when I felt the dreaded presence of death in my hospital room during January of 1973.

And throughout my illness I have been haunted with an overwhelming fear that my faith will not stand the final test.

Therefore, I need constant affirmation that I can make it — that God will see me through my toughest hour. If he doesn't, then those I love will question his reality. I feel this responsibility so strongly that the possibility of failure creates the deepest of all my fears. And with this is the fear that my very human depression will be interpreted by others as a lack of faith.

It has been so important to me to demonstrate the reality of Christ in my life that I will do almost anything to preserve that witness. But that has become increasingly difficult. Paul speaks of putting on the armor of faith.

There are big chinks developing in mine.

As the pain increases — so does this fear.

This fear has often virtually immobilized me. I find it difficult to accept my human condition. And the doubts I have about the reality of God, the life hereafter, and the validity of faith itself have become paralyzing. Is it possible that religion was invented to meet our needs? Will my disease make a cynic of me?

My dying would be easier if I could really believe there was an overall purpose for my life and death. But my pain and depression, and often my doubts, seem to keep me from believing that there is a creative power — a cosmic force — God using me for some purpose known only to him.

"Lord, thou bruises me, but since it's you, it's all right," said John Calvin.

In this context I have often thought of the meaning of redemption — to let God assume responsibility for my future — after I have done all I can. If I can trust God, then somehow out of my experience something good will come. It will be redeemed from nothingness to meaning so that my life will not have been in vain.

During the time that I was confronting some of the most critical questions about my personal faith, an incident occurred which impressed me deeply.

It was in the spring of 1974. Eunice Kronholm, a St. Paul banker's wife, was kidnapped and held seventy-two hours by her abductors.

Eunice is a member of the Mounds-Midway School of Nursing faculty. Although I do not know her well, I know she has a deep Christian faith. But I have found her story very difficult for me to accept.

She said her faith in God provided her with the inner resources to confront her personal ordeal. Why couldn't I find those inner resources — that presence of a personal God? I convinced myself that it was not so much her faith that gave her the resources, but the strength of her character and her own personality.

In facing death, I have often concluded that the only resource I had was my personal strength — which is waning and is increasingly less than I need in order to maintain my self-control and emotional balance. I often find myself with a spirit of desperation when my depression and lack of hope are in control.

There must be someone who can help me renew my faith. If only I can develop a close relationship with another person, maybe that will meet my need. Somehow I believe that person's strength and faith can be transferred to me.

And through it all there is Gordon, always assuring me he will be there — always wanting to provide that closeness I crave. Why can't he give that to me? And he replies, "Why don't you accept it?"

I have often thought of this as analogous to our concept of God's grace. It is freely given. All we need do is to be willing to accept. But our human desire to be independent makes it difficult, even impossible for some, to receive that gift.

The question of faith in conflict with humanity can never be resolved, I guess. Others seem to see that more clearly than I do. Maybe that's because their own thinking process has not been violated by drugs, which do strange things to me.

The Death of Jesus and the Stages of Dying

Dr. Elisabeth Kübler-Ross identifies five psychological stages in dying. In my search for a biblical faith to provide strength during my illness, I read and reread the account of Jesus' passion and death and discovered a parallel between Kübler-Ross's five stages and Jesus' final days (provided we begin from a premise which may be argued by some biblical scholars — that Jesus knew the ultimate consequence of his last journey to Jerusalem). Assuming that premise, let's take a look at Kübler-Ross's five steps — denial and isolation, anger, bargaining, depression, and acceptance.[2]

If Jesus didn't experience denial, there must have been some real

---

[2]Ibid., chapters 2-7

questions raised in his mind about his future when he rode trium-
phantly into Jerusalem on Palm Sunday. How could death — violent
death at that — be so close when he was affirmed by so many?

I find it difficult to believe that my own death is imminent on the days
when I feel good enough to do many of the things I really want to do.
And isn't my speaking, writing, and planning really a mechanism of
denial which helps me cope with my condition?

Isolation is also a part of this stage. In the Garden of Gethsemane,
following the last supper, three times Jesus begged his disciples to stay
with him. "My soul is very sorrowful, even to death; remain here and
watch with me" (Matthew 26:38). The loneliness, the isolation,
prompted him to waken them three times — to give him the comfort of
their presence, to fill the very human need of the presence of another
in a time of great crisis. He tried to get some kind of support from his
disciples, and all they did was sleep.

When it comes right down to it, you have to face this alone.

I have written of my own sense of aloneness — the feeling of
isolation which I anticipate will increase. As my illness progresses, my
sense of isolation increases. Aloneness is one of the worst of all human
experiences. And I have it day after day. Jesus could not overcome
that, and I find some understanding that if he couldn't, why should I
think I can span its abyss?

Some may argue that because of who Jesus was, he didn't experience Kübler-Ross's second stage in dying — anger. That's a very
human quality.

But my theology has become more human in the past few months
because I believe we have stressed a theology focusing on God and
the God in Christ. And we have neglected the man in Christ — a man
who felt as we feel. How can we fail to read anger into the words he
said to the women (Luke 23:29-30) who "bewailed and lamented
him" on his way to the cross? After he had stumbled under the load of
his own cross, and Simon the Cyrene was recruited to help, he turned
to the women and said:

Daughters of Jerusalem, do not weep for me, but weep for
yourselves and for your children. For behold, the days are
coming when they will say, "Blessed are the barren and the
wombs that never bore, and the breasts that never gave suck."
Then they will begin to say to the mountains, "Fall on us"; and
to the hills, "Cover us!"

Again, I can identify with that kind of anger — an emotion un-
leashed at doctors, nurses, clergy, my family — anyone near me. Not
because of who they are, but because of what is happening to me and

because they are escaping it, at least for now. I am angry because those whom I leave behind in my free-fall experience will remain and stay in their patterns and forms — and their life-type world.

I was so angry during my hospitalization following the liver biopsy that I have promised never to return to that nursing station. Every nurse there knows me, and I'm so ashamed of my violent reaction and rudeness that I don't want to face them any more. In the height of my pain and under medication, my personality changes — never for the best — and all my anger pours out on whoever is closest. Usually it was the nurse who experienced the focus of my anger. But if the doctor happened to come at those times, he took his lumps.

Bargaining is the third step in Kübler-Ross's stages of dying. The whole garden scene was, for Jesus, one of bargaining. The bargaining was so intense that the bargainer sweat drops like blood. When his bargaining wasn't accepted, he said, "Thy will be done. Nevertheless, not what I will, but what thou wilt" (See Mark 14:36).

With me it has not been a direct "I promise — if you only will," but the bargaining spirit has been there. I wanted to see my Paula graduate from high school; I want to see Gail achieve the same goal. And I want God to grant me that wish. In return I will at least be grateful, and at best I will use my time to be a better person.

As the Gospels record it, Jesus went through two stages almost simultaneously — bargaining (the third stage) and acceptance (the final or fifth stage of dying). The stages of dying are not necessarily chronological. In my own experience, I have moved back and forth through several of them a number of times. And there are those who never move out of one stage. I think of one who until the moment of her death never passed the denial stage. I'm sure there are many who can never allow their denial mechanism to go because that's the only way they can cope with the real prospect of death.

The fourth step is depression. "Why hast thou forsaken me?" said Jesus (Mark 15:34b). How depressed can one be then to feel abandoned even by God? It is difficult for me to believe that anyone faces death without the feeling that everyone has turned his back upon him — even God.

For me this has been the dominant stage — and I'm sure it is for many in prolonged illness. There is much to be depressed about. For one thing, I am greatly depressed by my appearance. I have gained almost seventy-five pounds since surgery in December, 1972. At one point I outgrew my clothes at the rate of two sizes a week! Now I am wearing a size twenty-two — a year ago, size fourteen. My head is bald, my joints swollen and ugly, and my body bloated — all caused

48

"Where are you going?"
Was the query, loud and firm.
"Where?" you ask. To a heaven of some kind.
Perhaps I am one of those
     who prefer falling.
     Falling asleep in the arms of Jesus.

This answer has a lot to offer
     you must admit.
Because it removes all the worry and doubt . . .
     and even the thinking about it all.

Asleep in the arms of Jesus
Yes, that is what we should tell them,
At least because it settles those unsettled feelings
     you have
And leads you straight to some good Heaven.

This just has to be some fabulous place
For Jesus himself will be there
And all will be just as we were taught.
Everything will be right as we thought.

Beautiful and lovely and secure . . .
You question this? How foolish.
Questions really get you nowhere
     except frustrated, frightened, and confused.
And there's enough of that stuff in this world anyway.

Yes, asleep in the arms of Jesus
"Safe on his gentle breast."
Asleep in the arms of Jesus —
That is sure security forevermore.

by my reaction to the use of chemotherapy. A depressing price for a woman to pay for such a limited life.

I was depressed when the full impact of my diagnosis hit me and again a year later when cancer was found in the bones, and once more I was prepared for death, only to respond favorably to a new drug and to hear Wayne say, "We have a partial remission." I was depressed to think of dying and sometimes equally as depressed to think of more of the kind of life I was living.

"Father, into thy hands I commit my spirit," represents Jesus in the final stage of death — acceptance (Luke 23:46). Although I have felt that spirit of acceptance, especially in the early stages of illness — it has been a long time since I have been willing to be accepting of my fate. I have verbalized it often, but I have not felt the peace that comes from the acceptance Jesus finally experienced.

That will come again, I am sure. When it does, the anger, depression, and rejection which I feel will be lost in the tenderness, forgiveness, and love that comes when any person accepts who he is and where he is. Then there is no need to prove anything — to fight back — to struggle for status or personhood. You have finally arrived. In that acceptance there will be peace — the peace for which I have longed in the restless months since I first learned I had terminal cancer.

The Biblical Record and Death

The Bible has also provided me with a resource to learn more about death itself. And it is not in the cliches we have been taught. After speaking to a class of seminary students, I was asked, "Don't you find hope in the promise you will fall asleep in the arms of Jesus?" My reply was, "I'd rather be awake!"

It wasn't until later that I thought that encounter seemed to be somewhat pornographic in its suggestiveness.

But this concept of death is supported and encouraged by the hymns we have been taught such as Fanny Crosby's "Safe in the Arms of Jesus."

I find little support for this concept in the Bible. I believe it is the product of our need for a sense of security and sureness in dealing with the afterlife. Maybe I would have been helped by straightforward, honest sermons about death. But I have missed them.

By avoiding such honesty about death, we Christians and our leaders deny the truth of the writer of Ecclesiastes, who reminds us there is "a time to be born, and a time to die . . ." (Ecclesiastes 3:2). Our greatest form of denial is to avoid this commonality we all share.

50

Safe in the arms of Jesus,
Safe on his gentle breast,
There by His love o'er-shaded,
Sweetly my soul shall rest.
Hark! 'tis the voice of angels,
Borne in a song to me,
Over the fields of glory,
Over the jasper sea . . .

Safe in the arms of Jesus,
Safe from corroding care,
Safe from the world's temptations,
Sin cannot harm me there.
Free from the blight of sorrow,
Free from my doubts and fears;
Only a few more trials,
Only a few more tears! . . .

Jesus, my heart's dear refuge,
Jesus has died for me;
Firm on the Rock of Ages,
Ever my trust shall be.
Here let me wait with patience,
Wait till the night is o'er;
Wait till I see the morning
Break on the golden shore . . .

CHORUS
Safe in the arms of Jesus,
Safe on His gentle breast,
There by His love o'ershaded,
Sweetly my soul shall rest.

I'm convinced most of us don't believe the New Testament, or death would have no fear. That's the paradox of my own experience. As a Christian, I believe death should have no fear for me.

But I don't want to die.

This life has been wonderful for me.

It's terrific.

I love it!

I'm not through.

I have lots of things to do.

It's distressing to know I won't be able to do them. Because there isn't time — or strength — or opportunity.

I don't understand why anyone would want to "blow out" of this life.

Therefore, I can't help asking: What is death? What follows? What is heaven? Is there such a place? Where is it? What does it mean? What is the life hereafter? Where am I going? What will it be like?

And I have raised these questions because I believe the pietism developed in the nineteenth century, encouraged by the hymns of Fanny Crosby and many of her contemporaries, has created a lot of garbage that has grown up about our ideas of heaven and eternal life. And it has been "dumped" on people by pietistic pastors and others in charge of religious thought — like, death is an easy passing — you'll come down a path and Jesus will take you by the hand to some never-never land where "you'll walk with Him and you'll talk with Him and. . . ."

How can we cut through those myths — the fantasies which we have been taught since Sunday School days about streets paved with gold and the cloud of witnesses we will join, especially as we live more and more in an astronaut-explored space? It just doesn't hold together.

I have missed theological insights that go beyond the biblical poetry of John and Paul, who try to describe the afterlife in words which their readers found expressed more feeling than reality.

It's much easier to deal with "streets of gold" and "rooms of a mansion" describing the afterlife than to deal with the resurrections

Death is so final.
So hard to understand.
The clues so few
  The feeling so new
    And final, too.

Death is something
That just doesn't happen
  Not to me, at least.
It happens to others far away
  But not to me at all, at all.

I shall go on forever
At least that's my hopeful plan.
I shall move steadily along and on
Toward some bright eternity.

Some bloodless, beautiful room, perhaps
Where perfection is everywhere.
That's the clue, the vital view
Of heaven; a rainbow hue.

Ivory palaces and golden streets
And a place of my very own.
Where I'll walk with him
  And talk with him
And live forevermore.

recorded in the New Testament. Why do we resort to such simplistic metaphors? Because the resurrection accounts in the New Testament have little information to offer.

There are three miracles recorded in the Gospels which tell of Jesus raising people from the dead — the widow's son at Nain (Luke 7:11-17), the daughter of Jairus (Mark 5:22-24, 35-43; Luke 8:40-42, 49-56), and Lazarus (John 11:1-44). The Gospel writers are silent as to what the subjects experienced from the time of their death until Jesus restored their life.

There are a variety of reasons offered for this. In Lazarus's case, some have suggested he was dumb and couldn't speak, which may account for John's failure to record what happened to Lazarus in death. Since John had a unique interest in people, he gives us the best insight of all the Gospel writers into the people with whom Jesus came in contact. For that reason his silence about Lazarus is significant.

But all that is recorded is that "Lazarus came forth." No clues are given as to what he experienced.

The other two events were recorded by Mark and Luke, whose basic interest is always centered in the life and ministry of Jesus. For that reason, according to biblical scholars, they were not interested in the experience during death, but rather the fact that Jesus performed a miracle. That was what they wanted recorded.

The Bible also fails to record any description from Jesus following the three days in the tomb. And there are no words from those whose graves were opened during the dramatic experiences recorded during the terror of the crucifixion — when the temple veil was torn asunder, the sky became black, the winds blew, and the graves were opened.

In discussing this with Grandfather, he kept pressing me about the unwritten clues. "Why aren't there any," he kept asking me, "if we are supposed to know?" He said when you read about death in the New Testament, "Look not only for what is written, but also for that which is omitted."

There are a variety of reasons suggested for the biblical silence about these who were raised from the dead by Jesus.

David Bartlett, pastor of the University Baptist Church in Minneapolis, Minnesota, has helped me to think through many of the questions I have about the biblical concept of death and resurrection. He suggests that one reason for silence is that the early Judeo-Christian concept of death was that of falling asleep and that the dead would be awakened at the Last Judgment. Therefore, the death experience offered nothing to report. The idea that people go to be with God, David reminded me, didn't come into the tradition until

Luke's and maybe John's Gospels.

Furthermore, David points out, the Gospel writers recorded the resurrection stories not as reporters but as those interested in writing down oral tradition which had been honed and sharpened to focus exclusively on Jesus.

David helped me to see that the New Testament focus for all miracles is always on Jesus and the response of faith to him. Therefore, blind people don't talk about what it's like to be blind, the deaf about being deaf, or demoniacs about what it's like to be possessed. But it sure would have helped us if one of those resurrected could have given us some clue about what it felt like in the life beyond death.

But I can't escape the conclusion that the purpose of the resurrection experiences was not to give us clues into the afterlife, but to affirm the power of Jesus to make life new NOW.

What was Jesus here for? What was his death supposed to say? What part did his death play? Jesus' death tells us why he lived. His experience centers in the reality that life and death really are of one piece.

None of us lives to himself, and none of us dies to himself. If we live, we live to the Lord, and if we die, we die to the Lord; so then, whether we live or whether we die, we are the Lord's. For to this end Christ died and lived again, that he might be Lord both of the dead and of the living (Romans 14:7-9).

Eternal life in the New Testament refers to one piece. It is not futuristic, in the "sweet bye and bye," but refers to the quality of life Jesus gives us now and which is sustained beyond physical death. It becomes real in our "new birth" and continues to grow and develop from that point of decision in this life into the enrichment of life that follows our earthly existence.

I have shared with people my conclusion that "In my house there are many mansions — I have a nice room ready for you" is simply a poetic way of expressing something that is so wonderful and beyond us that we just don't know a more adequate medium to explain it. By poetry, men throughout history have described ideas which were limited by the use of words. The terms used are descriptive myths.

So they are for me.

You die your way.

Me — I'm not at all worried about whether or not there's a mansion in heaven for me or whether that was just a beautiful term to describe whatever's coming after this. And I believe that's going to be great.

But that belief doesn't remove my fear of death.

I don't mind telling anyone that I'm afraid to die. I firmly believe everyone is afraid — with perhaps the exception of the aged, whose bodies have deteriorated to the point where death is welcome. I don't believe those who tell me, "If God calls me tomorrow, I won't be afraid to die."

> **Lord,**
> **If I have to die,**
> **Let me die;**
> **But please,**
> **Take away this fear.**
> **— Ken Walsh**[3]

To fear death doesn't make me less of a Christian.

It affirms my humanity.

But most of us are afraid of any new experience because we fear the unknown.

I have a better chance to adjust to a new experience if I have a few clues as to what to expect. But there are very few to guide us in death. We just say to God, "I'm yours."

Metaphysically I find some support for my belief that our existence will be different. In some cultures prior to our technological age, death was similar to the transition from spring to winter. Like Jonathan Livingston Seagull, it is the passage to life at a higher level.

A sermon sent to me by a minister friend points out to us that nature offers many illustrations of this — the seed that becomes a plant, the polliwog that becomes a frog, the caterpillar that becomes a butterfly. The frog is no longer dependent upon life in the water as he once was. The butterfly is no longer confined to crawling along a surface, but enters a new dimension.

And our own birth from our mother's womb is the traumatic experience in human existence when we are physically transformed into an entirely different dimension of life. We are freed to a new life, shedding the placenta and the cord to begin life in a new dimension.

And as great as this life has been for me, my faith is that whatever God has in store for me will be better. It's a leap of faith I take from this life to the next.

---

[3] Ken Walsh, *Sometimes I Weep* (Valley Forge: Judson Press, 1974), p. 18. Copyright © S.C.M. Press Ltd.

Following a visit in my hospital room, a Roman Catholic priest left this prayer by Thomas Merton:

My Lord God, I have no idea where I am going. I do not see the road ahead of me. I cannot know for certain where it will end. Nor do I really know myself, and the fact that I think that I am following your will does not mean that I am actually doing so. But I believe that the desire to please you does in fact please you. And I hope I have that desire in all that I am doing. I hope that I will never do anything apart from that desire. And I know that if I do this you will lead me by the right road, though I may know nothing about it. Therefore I will trust you always though I may seem to be lost and in the shadow of death. I will not fear, for you are ever with me, and you will never leave me to face my perils alone.[4]

I find hope, not in the poetry or in the limited dissertations on death in the Scriptures, nor in metaphysical arguments, but in the affirmation that God is real and that he has not created us for waste. I am convinced that the eternal quality of our life that sets us apart from all other living creatures will go on beyond the limitations we have experienced as humans.

Although I have found little help from the Scriptures to tell me what my life after death will be, I know it will be different. Even as the resurrected Jesus had changed so that he was not readily identified — so it will be with me.

For me, that belief is a leap of faith.

The first leap I made was to give my life to God in this present life. That was an act of faith. And when you decide you are going to be God's person and not your own, you really don't know where that is going to take you or what you are going to do or where you are going to be. It's a leap of faith.

Dying, in my best understanding after these many months, is that time when I take my second leap of faith. It's a part of the free fall — like the trapeze artist high above the crowd who suddenly falls. And seemingly from nowhere with split-second timing, his partner below swings out, reaches out, catches him, and saves him.

That leap of faith is when I take my last conscious breath. In faith, I believe God will reach out and catch me.

[4] Thomas Merton, *Thoughts in Solitude* (New York: Farrar, Straus & Giroux, Inc., 1958), p. 83. Reprinted by permission of Farrar, Straus & Giroux, Inc. Copyright © 1956, 1958, by the Abbey of Our Lady of Gethsemani.

In faith I believe it.

In faith I believe that the God who has been faithful, just, and the one whom I have trusted all my life will be there. I will become a different kind of God-person. I don't know what that means, for sure, nor does anyone.

It's one of the great risks of human experience. And as Jesus took that risk, not knowing what was coming after, so do we — "into Thy hands I commit my spirit."

God has not deserted me in life. Neither will he in death. And I have confidence he knows the way. I'm apprehensive and often frightened, but just as I have taken the leap of faith before, I'm prepared for this one. I believe that whatever God has in store for me, as his person, it will be better than the life I've enjoyed here — great as that has been.

> The leap of faith
> To what destination—
> A place so high
> In some ethereal sky.
> Bye - bye!
> Some say so.

Out of the Second World War comes the story of a father and his daughter seeking refuge from the bombs that showered London. He found a deep crater, which he thought would offer safety and took shelter there. He called to his daughter, telling her to jump. She was afraid of the darkness below and said, "But I can't see you." And he replied, "It's all right — I can see you." So she jumped and was caught in his waiting arms. We can't see God waiting for us. But he can see us.

That's the leap of faith.

During my hospitalization in January and February, 1973, I asked John Sundquist, at the conclusion of a visit one day, to come back in two days prepared to recite everything he could remember that the Bible had to say about resurrection.

When he returned, I said, "OK, John, what can you say?"

John replied, "JoAnn, anything I can say you already know. You know the data as well as I do — if not better. So we can have a sword drill on Scripture about resurrection, and we might fight to a draw. Instead, why don't we talk about it like we do in Agora — and tell each other where we really are. Say it, JoAnn — where are you in your own faith and belief about Jesus Christ?"

I replied, "Well, John — that's it, that's where it's really at — that's where it is and always has been."

John said, "And that's your hope."

The astronauts have gone so high
And leaped about on the moon.
But all we found there were rocks and the like—
No God; for he had already gone to some sweet bye and bye.
He wasn't there, and there was no palace at all—
Yet some still cling to such
      With hope.

Maybe He is a She
Or a combination of the two.
Perhaps our God is sexless
Dwelling on far more important issues
   than masculinity.
      Do you suppose?
      I sure hope so.

Then his word "children of God"
Will burst into clear focus
And we will see at the end
   of this leap of faith
The freedom and joy of a little child.

"Do you really believe it?" I asked.

"Yes, I do," he said.

"Then I guess I do, too," I replied.

John continued, "As corny as it sounds, JoAnn, our hope is found in the first Bible verse you ever learned."

I didn't understand what he meant so he quoted John 3:16: "For God so loved the world that he gave his only Son, that whoever believes in him should not perish. . . ."

And then he said, "We know that God comes in history; we have the biblical record of Israel; the historical event of Jesus Christ; and we know when his spirit touches ours. And that God who initiates the action brings it to completion. God who brings us to birth continues to be with us. It is terrible to conceive that God would bring us to this point — then annihilation."

Then I said, "I wish Brian could believe it just isn't a hoax."

John put his arms around me and hugged me tightly and said, "As your priest, I assure you of your forgiveness. You are somebody. You are accepted — and he is with you now and ever will be."

"I believe it," I replied.

Then I said,: "Funny thing — I know when it's all over that it will be a great experience, but darn it, there are some pretty great experiences I'd still like to have here."

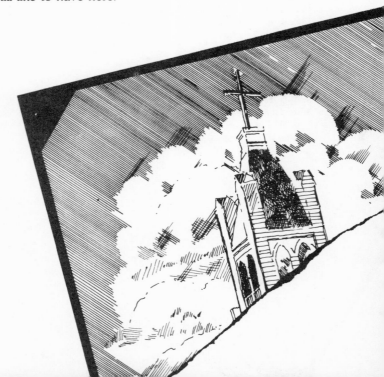

"Maybe I would have been helped by straight-forward, honest sermons about death. But I have missed them."

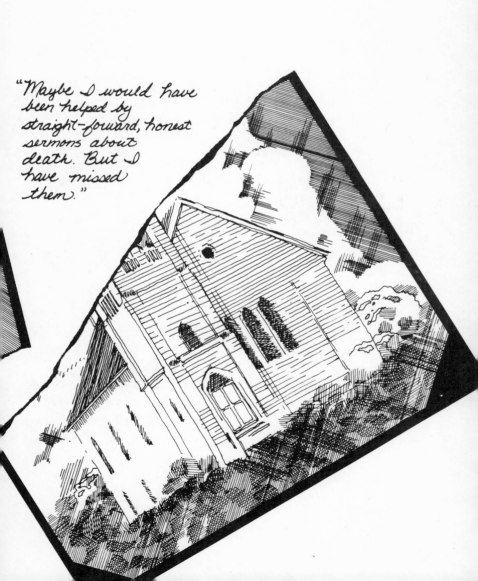

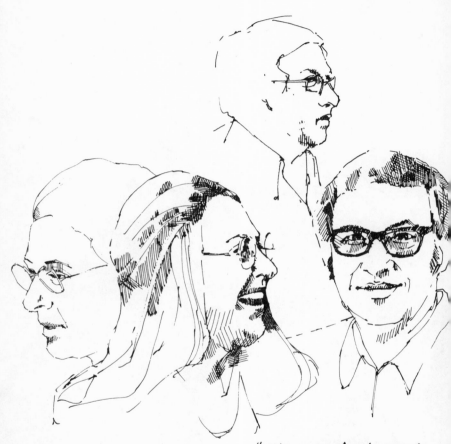

"It's very hard now to keep the reality of death before us when you are doing so well."

During the time I was home for Christmas in 1972 I made plans for what I believed to be an imminent death. That preparation for death would symbolize the reality of my separation and would make the free fall more real for us all. I made peace with my family and with them I outlined my memorial service. I said good-bye to dear friends and extracted promises that they would never leave me no matter what happened. I even secured from Gordon the promise that he would not remarry until Gail finished high school. In a way, I had planned when and how I would die.

But God spoiled my plans.

Death did not come as I expected.

My recovery following surgery December 28, 1972, was good, and on January 18, 1973, I was discharged from the hospital because Wayne felt I would "do better at home." However, I continued to weaken and was without an appetite. So on January 28, I was readmitted to begin my chemotherapy treatments.

My reaction to the first two treatments was not good. I was growing weaker and felt the end was near. Out of sheer exhaustion and apathy I was giving up.

After the second treatment Wayne told Gordon, "If JoAnn fails to respond, we'll stop treatment — I don't believe in shooting a person full of chemicals if we don't get a positive reaction."

And then it happened. I began to lose my hair. Sores developed in my mouth. I was nauseated. I felt even worse than before, and the strange thing was — Wayne was noticeably pleased!

The pack of five chemicals known as Cooper's Regimen fed intravenously and supplemented orally was doing its work. He explained that the chemicals killed the fastest growing cells in the body — among them, those in the scalp and in the mouth, but also, and more importantly, the deadly cancer cells. In a few days I was ready to go home again. My appetite and strength had returned, so I was discharged on February 27. I'm sure Wayne felt it wouldn't be long before I'd be back, but that wasn't the way it would be.

I had a whole year and a new vocation to pursue before I would be back in the hospital.

When I returned home, a letter from an old friend, a professional educator for twenty-five years was waiting for me. He wrote:

I know that I was born both to live and to die. My problem is to accept the fact that the time is not really within my control. Perhaps you have an advantage at this point. I have come to the conclusion that learning how to die is as important as learning to live. As one who has been related to education for a long while, you may well be doing the most important teaching of your whole life. I hope that each of us may learn from you. We will bless you for your helpfulness.

That gave me the encouragement I needed to use my experience as a learning opportunity for all those with whom I came in contact. I readied myself to enter this new phase of my life.

My new vocation began a few weeks later, in March, 1973, when I was asked to speak to the nursing students at Mounds-Midway School of Nursing in St. Paul. A sensitive young reporter, Brian Anderson, was there and wrote up my story, which appeared on the front page of the April 13 issue of the *Minneapolis Tribune*. This opened many doors for me, and soon I was speaking on an average of twice a week before audiences in schools, churches, civic clubs, hospitals, and professional nursing organizations.

I felt that my mission was to help people understand death by sharing with them the honest feelings I had about what was happening to me. I firmly believed that if I had a better understanding of death, I could confront my own experience better. But it has only been the experiences of the intervening months since I learned I had terminal cancer that have caused me to do the hard thinking every human must do if death is to be confronted creatively.

Death is something we are more prone to think about when we are young. For example, many young people I know talk about their premonitions of death and write stories or poems about death. Brian has written and had published several poems, about half of them concerning death.

I suspect that the reason for this is that when death seems far away it is easier to contemplate. In a sense it is fantasy — play-acting. In our youth we assume there will be many tomorrows. But the older we get the more we realize there will be an end of tomorrows as our yesterdays stretch farther and farther behind us. Yet the inevitability of death somehow doesn't apply to us.

In the summer of 1973, when I was feeling fairly well, Gordon and I again went to a lakeside cottage up north for a week to recuperate from the emotional buildup we were experiencing at home. I was feeling so much better — and was able to deal with most everything that came along — and I shall always remember his saying, "It's very hard now, isn't it, to keep the reality of death before us when you are doing so well?"

But death doesn't die. It is real.

Grandfather asked me, "Would you have been as interested as you are in learning about death if you were not dying?" The answer was and is obvious. Since then I have given a great deal of thought to that question. "Everyone should think about his own death at least once a day," someone suggested to me.

And that's good advice.

Each day would be a lot different.

There is a fine line between being obsessed by the thought of death and living with it as an ever-present reality — not to be feared, but to be affirmed. A friend said to me, "We cannot make sense of our lives unless we can make sense out of our death." This is the context for contemplating death daily, that is, to give life a center of meaning — real meaning. It's not that one thinks, "I want a bronze coffin. . . ." It is rather, "How's my life going?" or "If I don't have too much time left, what do I want to do with it?" Dealing with the reality of death makes a difference in the way we live.

For me, living with death as an ever-present reality is an experience in death education and prepares me for the inevitable. So I try to communicate the value of my new life-style — a style which tends to remove the paralyzing fear of the unknown and frees a person to enjoy life now.

Living with that awareness makes life more valuable — not less; more meaningful — not more depressing; richer — not poorer.

Most of us act like a child in the dark when we talk of death. To dispel that fear, we turn on the light. I believe that death education is the light we turn on to remove part of the fear of death. That light simply is an awareness of death's reality and the acknowledgment that we can't escape it.

This awareness helps us examine and understand our own feelings about death. Therefore, part of the teaching mission to which I have given the balance of my life is to prod people into thinking about their own attitudes toward death. Are they motivated by anger towards God so they would curse out against him, or by professionalism, piety, or self-pity? Or are they motivated by an acceptance of death as one of the natural events of our human destiny?

But to participate in any kind of death education requires openness on the part of both the teacher and the learner.

It was in this spirit that the teacher of our youngest daughter, Gail, approached her and asked her to write a story relating her feelings, and that of our family, in this experience. She called the story "The Promised Beginning — Life." She wrote:

The promised new beginning of another day
Wondering of its likeness,
Hoping it will always stay.
Sitting by myself in the room
Letting the sun shine through
Wishing a day like this
Will come again soon.
Will tomorrow be different?
Will I be changed?
Will everybody seem strange?
Will I cope?
All I can do is pray and hope.

By helping her to deal openly with her personal feelings, an understanding teacher helped Gail learn the meaning of the death experience. And the value Gail placed on the experience is found at the end of the story, which she closed with, "Death is life's exclamation point," a quotation she remembered reading somewhere.

Gail's teacher perceived death education as offering the positive value of anticipatory grief, which each member of our family has experienced. This has given them the opportunity to express their love, care, and concern for me. And in their own way all the members of the family have expressed their love for me. We have remembered the good times we've had together — and we have cried together.

Anticipatory grief will not relieve them from all the pain which they will feel when separation is final. And I hope my life has meant enough that there will be some sense of loneliness in those whose life and love I have shared so deeply. But it is made easier because we have all had time to work it through, and the actual crisis of death will be lessened. That has happened only because our family faced death openly and dealt with our feelings honestly, not once but many times. Gordon and our children have wept tears of grief so often in these long months that I really believe grieving will give way to celebration when this ordeal is over.

As for me, anticipatory grief has been one of the most affirming emotions I have experienced in these long months. It would be untrue to say that I have not felt deep sadness and have also experienced grief over the prospect of separation. But to know I have been loved deeply enough to cause others to grieve has kept me from feeling totally bitter — and often lessened the feeling of aloneness.

I will remember until that part of me dies the deep impression made on me by the mature men in my life who freely showed their emotions when they first saw me after the terminal diagnosis was known. They were open in their physical expressions of love — based on that special depth of feeling one human can experience for another. And together we grieved in anticipation of the final separation.

But our openness in this experience has caused some embarrassment and risk. We discovered that our frank way of discussing our situation created a lot of probing into the privacy of our lives. There was the young nursing student who, during a question and answer period following a presentation we had made, asked Gordon how illness had affected our sex life!

When the article appeared in the Minneapolis Tribune, Gordon was called by a very hostile, elderly man who offered his sympathy because I had stated that in the death experience I was growing farther and farther away from my family. He took exception to the feeling of separation and loneliness which I find growing each day. He said that his wife had died a few weeks earlier and that during her final illness they had grown closer to each other than at any point in their long marriage.

And there was the pastor who also expressed his hostility toward me because he heard me openly speak of my doubts and fears regarding my faith and the life hereafter. His response was, "I would never express my concern to her by writing or speaking to her personally."

I came to accept this hostility as expressions of those who fail to understand my own humanness in resenting the fact that I am dying while others live.

And there was another friend who expressed his anger, as several have done, over my "flippancy" in dealing with death in an open and often humorous way.

But at the other extreme were people like Lynne, one of our foster daughters, who came to talk to me after she learned I was going to die. She expressed a feeling which others have stated in different ways by saying, "You seem to be something special now — like a superhuman person. You have super strength and insight." Others have asked me to support them, build them up, and make this experience easier for them.

From the very beginning I have feared that my openness would lead to making this experience a super ego-trip. To have people believe that because I can discuss what is happening to me I possess unusual insight or power feeds my ego.

This has led to one of the greatest temptations I face in this experience — that of sainthood. I am often tempted by those who believe I now can do something special for them. To yield to this temptation would make me one of the greatest manipulators of all. By using the high emotions created in this experience and touching the feelings now open to me, I can get people to do things for me and use them for almost any purpose. And this temptation to act as a superhuman lends itself to the idea that I can be some kind of saint — acting and doing like no one else — here and in eternity.

I was awed by John Burns' request to ask God to make a place for him and by Rita's plea to intervene on her behalf so that she would be a better mother and wife and be assured of God's presence in eternity.

But I have been turned off by many others who have sought identification with me so that I could say hello to Grandma, or to their child. "Tell them I'll be there soon," one said. And another, "Greet my wife for me."

To be alone
   is the most desperate state of mind.
Alone, not lonely,
For that we seldom are.

There are always folks coming and going
   with cheery greetings and baskets of chicken
      to lose it all.

But words and food don't fill the gap,
   that enormous flap,
      open to that unknown.

To be alone is to be forsaken,
   a kind of leper-person
For in dying one becomes undesirable
And this aloneness is unshared.

To be lonely is just to be separated
From relationships pleasing and pleasant.
And loneliness can be altered
By reforming or repairing a place in the group.

In death one is so alone,
The most devastating of situations.
A want for sharing is ever desired
But when leaving behind this flesh and bone
One goes alone.

The list of favors I've been asked to do is very long. But since God works in the twinkling of an eye, I'm sure he'll have time to deal with them.

Even though I don't believe I can honor these requests, I have felt the emotional responsibility laid on me — and it's enormous. That's a really heavy load for a dying person who's trying like everything to hang on. What do I say? I can't say no. So I say, "Well, I'll do my best."

But, theologically, I know this responsibility is not mine to assume. Each of us must work out his own salvation — to deny that is to deny one's personal responsibility — one's very personhood.

I cannot help people as they expect me to do and give them the one thing we all seek — hope.

Nevertheless, I have great difficulty dealing with those who have such high expectations of me because somehow they feel I am closer than they are to God and to things of eternal value and worth. Is that why some people, including my children, have felt the need to confess? For others, the need to set things right?

I have tried to share honestly with people the emotions I have experienced during my illness. This has not been easy for many reasons. Honesty is often misunderstood, and I fear the judgment of people who may disagree with me. Honesty can often hurt people — including the one who is being honest. But it has also been difficult because my emotions are in conflict and often ambivalent.

Furthermore, the emotional impact of a relatively quick death may be quite different from what my family and I are experiencing in prolonged illness. I have had almost two years for my emotions to intensify — and to change. So the climate of our family in crisis may be very different from that of another's.

Crisis infers an immediate problem which requires action now to resolve that difficulty — like the relationship between a husband and wife which has deteriorated to the point that some immediate decisions and actions are required to preserve or dissolve the marriage and/or protect the children. No matter how serious our personal crisis is, most of us can handle the short-term emotional trauma it creates.

But prolonged illness which creates a prolonged crisis is another problem.

After the liver biopsy, Gordon asked the surgeon, "How much time?" And he replied as only a responsible physician could, "I don't know — but we're not talking about years — only months." Those months have dragged into years due to successful chemotherapy, creating the crisis of prolonged illness. That has got to be a special kind of hell. It has been for me anyway. That's why I have such a tough time with those who say, "Take each day at a time," for each day seems worse than the last.

Gordon and I and our family — like others in similar circumstances — are going through one of the toughest, most demanding physical, emotional, and spiritual experiences that humans are called upon to do. And it never stops.

Several of our friends and acquaintances have died since my diagnosis, more than I care to count. Some suddenly. Others with only a short time to prepare.

My sister often says what others have said in one way or another, "I could walk off the curb today and be killed by a car." And that's true. Sudden death happened to a close friend or ours while I was still recuperating from the liver biopsy. He was a doctor, in excellent health — killed instantly in an auto accident.

But the difference is that the victim of sudden death does not have to think about it every day for months on end. He has been spared the long-term consciousness and anxiety of a prolonged death. Every day I have pain, and every day I think of how much worse it will get. I think of Gail — will her life be altered for good or bad without a mother to help guide her through her last two years of high school? I think of Paula, whose strong Christian motivation has always been to serve the undesirables of our society, and I wonder if the immense responsibility she shared with her dad during her sixteenth year, running our large home, will change her significantly in the years ahead? What do premature expectations do to the growing-up process of a strong girl like her?

I think of Gordon and what he will do.

I wonder what the shock of death will be like and what's beyond.

My mind never strays from the fear, apprehension — the uncertainty of tomorrow.

And there seems little to hope for.

71

Gordon and I have often talked about which is the better way to go. He says if he can't take it with him — he's not going! But we all *are*. And I believe prolonged illness is far more destructive to the person dying and for those around them than sudden death. This may not be true for everyone, for we have had calls from surviving mates telling us that the time they had together from the first knowledge of terminal illness until the end was the richest of their life together. But I suspect that more will identify with where we are in our experience.

For one thing, people expect more of me because, they say, "you look so good," and they tell me what I ought to do. When I respond with, "I haven't the strength or the motivation," they can't understand. I believe they go away feeling "she's just being stubborn and trying to get my sympathy."

I feel judged by them. They make me feel that I am shirking responsibilities. They have not accepted the fact that I have a mass in me that is draining my energy and will soon kill me.

Not only have I lost the strength to do what I would like to do, but I have also lost my emotional stability as well and find myself acting contrary to my true feelings. For example, during my illness I frequently reject Brian, whom I love very much, and make him leave the house because he takes issue with me and is confrontive. And Gail's diary recorded an experience in the hospital when I turned my back on her and refused her comfort and support. She wrote, "I had the worst feeling of rejection I've ever experienced." When she and her father got into the car to return home, she wrote, "I let all my feelings go." I love Gail and would never treat her that way — except for my disease.

And this simply illustrates the emotional confusion of a dying person. I'm not sure why, but I want to accept, and I end up rejecting; I want to love but often show hostility; I find peace but am often afraid; I am willing to surrender but more often seek to control; I seek joy and find sadness; and I have a faith but live with insecurity.

And there *is* pain, but it isn't the pain as much as it is the emotional instability which is my partner in prolonged illness. Pain only bothers *me*. But my emotions take their toll on everyone near me.

During the long months of my illness, I have often lost control of my emotions. And a person controlled by emotions can never be rational. So that's why it's difficult for people to relate to me — and me to them. It can be done only as we get in touch with each other's feelings. And mine are so wrapped up in where I am that it's almost impossible for those who love me the most to understand me — so that Gail asks her father, "How many times do we have to adjust?" Nobody can really predict how I will relate to another on a particular day.

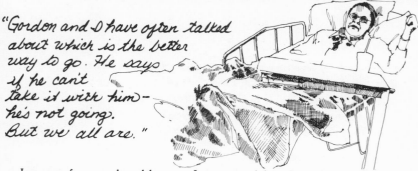

"Gordon and I have often talked about which is the better way to go. He says if he can't take it with him — he's not going. But we all are."

In one of my early addresses, I expressed fear for the personality change that drugs would induce. I feared becoming ugly, irritable, and unkind. This is a heavy responsibility for one in prolonged illness. The family will soon get over whatever hardships this experience creates. But I will lose my life. And my memory may be stained by the person which has been created by my disease.

When I first knew I was going to die, I was very angry. But soon I worked through that and became open and more loving. I found a certain peace in my relationships with others. All was in order. I hoped for more time but wasn't sure why, as bad as I felt. So I was prepared to die.

In the months since then I have rarely had that same accepting spirit of readiness. On the one hand, I am afraid to die, but on the other hand, I want to be released.

I often reject people, and that is easy to do for they set themselves up for my rejection. My depression and hostility make it easy for my family to find cause to confront me. And when they do, it becomes a personal affront and I reject them. I find it impossible to accept confrontation because no one should take issue with a dying person. I tell myself, "How cruel! How could they question me?" With them I often use the worn-out "You'll be sorry when I'm gone."

The desire to build a sense of guilt into those closest to me for not treating me the way I feel they should is often unconscious — but real.

The heavy responsibility of dealing with so many problems of my foster teenagers and that of keeping our big home often cause me to beg to leave — or at least have more help. And under that pressure, Gordon weakens and begins to make plans to remove ourselves from our mission.

But then I know I can't leave the house I love and all the things to which I have such an emotional and sentimental attachment, nor can I share my control over it or the children. So life continues in tension — a tension I know will exist no matter where I live — for the tension between the desire for less responsibility and the need to be needed will go with me wherever I live out my last days. At least this way my mood swings; and depression, despair, and rejection find difficulty in focusing on twelve moving targets, rather than only on the four of my immediate family. And Gordon perceives that better than I.

The emotional conflicts can be blamed partly on the drugs. They often create a euphoria which makes me feel good and causes hyperactivity. That will surely lead to a "down." And each one is lower than the one before. When it comes, all the negative emotional feelings take control.

This is particularly true in my relationship with Gordon. He has great difficulty in coping with my emotional swings. To preserve his own balance he often leaves the room, especially when I vent my anger and hostility. He tells me, "I love you, but I can't take it any longer. I will be in the house if you need me — but I won't remain in this room."

He deals with his anxiety by working compulsively. For example, he loses himself in the many projects to be done in the house until finally he drops into bed and immediate sleep, sometimes while I am still pouring out my angry feelings at him and the world he can cope with — but I cannot.

And when I was hospitalized, following my last surgery, he and some friends completely re-did our bedroom. Through his compulsiveness, he tries to keep himself together. That's also how he copes with his grief.

I have never really been convinced that he understands how much it hurts me to see him do all the things we used to do together but now I can no longer do. I resent his energy and zest for life. I resent the fact that he will live and do the things I had hoped and dreamed we would do together. And it doesn't help for him to remind me that life without me will create problems for him that he feels will be insurmountable.

Gordon is a strong person and he has a clearly defined theological base from which he operates. But this experience has been very hard on him. Sometimes I think it bothers him more than me — he's overanxious. For example, if I don't call him in the morning, he starts to fret, and if I fail to call in the afternoon, he gets nervous. So he works out his anxieties physically, and I worry that he will work himself into something he can't control.

I am concerned over his preoccupation with our crisis, often evidenced by his staring into space and his inability to concentrate when the young people in our home or I discuss a problem with him. I worry over his lapses of memory and his emotional exhaustion. In some ways he has lost touch with reality and returns only when he is shocked back through new experiences at home or at work.

Our relationship is tested by how we try to confront problems. With each problem he has to decide, "Shall I discuss this with her?" If he doesn't, I become angry. If he does, I avoid coping with it.

It's very hard on him because we have always gone a lot and done a lot. Now we don't. Life has become a drag. It *is* a drag to have a sick person around — for months.

When we do go, I find little joy unless the experience somehow centers around my needs and concerns. Otherwise I'm bored. And when I am, the evening is a failure for both of us. I strongly identify with Stewart Alsop, who found the support he needed from one physician because their conversation always centered around Mr. Alsop.

At times I have great guilt feelings about what my death will do to Gordon. He will be left with a twenty-one-room house for which there is a limited market. He will be left with the enormous emotional and financial burdens that I intended to share with him. He will have the sole responsibility for being mother and father to six foster children. The care of the house alone is a full-time job, and the emotional drain and demands of six problem teenagers seem to overwhelm him. Also to be able to carry off the mission of our home requires income from his work.

We often talk of our mission to our foster children, and I have asked Gordon many times, "What is happening to our dream?" We had committed ourselves to that ministry for ten years, feeling that in that period of our life we would have the most to offer those who were sent to us by the courts. After that, we would have fulfilled a mission for others and would be ready for a quieter life together.

But during the months of my illness our dream often fades.

It is increasingly difficult for me to cope with the emotional charge of our house. I am not "together" much of the time and therefore am unable to help the young people who come to "get it together" for themselves. I am unable to do the hard physical work of the house, which places an extra burden on Gordon, Paula, and Gail. Gordon often has to take up work that I leave undone because I am too sick to do it. And there is the increasing financial drain because of the need to employ help to share the responsibilities of the home.

When the emotional strain becomes almost unbearable — when we become exhausted by the time demands, such as picking up one of our teenagers at some police station in the middle of the night or talking with them until early in the morning to work through a problem that requires immediate attention — we seriously discuss leaving our home.

And in those times our dream becomes a nightmare.

But our deep financial commitment and the inadvisability of making any change while my future is so uncertain stop us short.

The guilt feelings I have about leaving Gordon with so much responsibility often are replaced by deep resentment. In those times I tell myself that he will begin a new life. And because he will have that opportunity, I find myself resentful.

I will not allow an in-depth discussion of this or any problem he tries to share with me because I find myself drifting farther away from him. Our relationship has slowly deteriorated.

Before my illness, we often showed our love in a variety of physical ways. But my response gradually waned, and I often want no part of a physical relationship with him. I feel I have to forfeit any intimacy. I reject his advances and even his attempts to kiss me good-bye when he leaves for work in the morning. I just can't be responsive.

His mere presence reminds me that he is a living person and that I am dying. And I become more comfortable when he is gone.

While I separate myself farther and farther from Gordon, my need for a physical relationship is met by friends whom I love, kiss, and touch. At one point I moved into a bedroom on the third floor and found myself escaping there whenever Gordon was getting too close to where I was emotionally. I have my defenses up and am determined that no one will break through to discover my greatest fears and insecurities.

But the strange paradox is that I want that closeness now more than ever. And the more I seek it the farther away I drive those who can give it to me.

Gordon reacts to this with obvious anxiety, but continues to assure me he understands and will stand by to the end no matter what I do.

Gordon and I have often talked about the concept of an open marriage. Since I have been sick, I have verbalized to groups my wish that Gordon felt free to develop relationships with other women. That would help meet some of his emotional needs. I'm not sure I could handle that. But if I could, I'm sure it would be best for him.

During a meeting of Agora I suggested to a small group of friends that a religious community should affirm the emotional separation which occurs between mates in prolonged illness. The mate who is well should be encouraged to develop normal and supportive relationships with members of the opposite sex. That would be a healthy way for Gordon to face his future.

How vividly I can remember the long hours Gordon and I often spent on Sunday evenings, often until 2:00 A.M., trying to "put together" one of our foster girls after a weekend with her parents. It was several months before the alienation that had developed between her and her parents over several years was removed. When she was able to break the emotional ties with her parents, was ready to take responsibility for her own life — to become independent — she could become the person she wanted to be.

In the same way Gordon needs to establish emotional independence from me. He has been drained in meeting my needs, and only as he begins to separate himself from me will he be able to find someone to replenish these needs.

My own children have helped me understand this as they have tried to convince me that even Gordon is human and his emotional needs are just as real as mine. And they remain unmet. Although he tells me he will stay by me, I often wonder when and if his personal resources and patience will be exhausted. For example, his anger often rises until he becomes short-tempered with everybody.

His preoccupation with attempts to handle me cause both frustration in his work and errors in judgment dealing with critical problems of our home. His usual logical and objective way of coping with everyday problems is impaired and often gives way to rationalizing things he would never do except for the pressure of our crisis.

At the age of forty-seven his sex drives continue to be normal. Mine are gone. Gail and Paula sense his vulnerability and become over-protective of any kind of contact he has with women, often our mutual friends. He assures me even though that part of our relationship is over, the depth of love he has for me has not diminished. But our sexual relationship has always been an important part of our marriage, and because its mutual enjoyment is gone, I now realize death has come to another area of human existence that made life so good for me. It is lost in my free fall. This has become another source of my deep depression.

There is his constant plea to avoid the danger of self-fulfilling prophecy. He says that to remind him that he is not the one who can give me the support I need — to reiterate "you are a rotten person" — will, in fact, make him one. And the same is true of each of our children and our foster children. I see it happening but often can't control it.

In terms of transactional analysis, my attempt to be an "OK" person makes it necessary to put others down. "I'm OK" because they are "not OK."

We both find it difficult to affirm each other. With our friends, we can say yes. But in the intimacy of marriage we are losing this. I guess this is because I am unable somehow to involve him in the emotional struggles through which I am going. This is a new dimension in our marriage, for our relationship has always been open. Together we were able to cope with all kinds of problems.

77

In spite of our strong personalities, we could usually work towards a mutually agreeable solution without sacrificing our personal integrity. Our problem solving involved emotional upheavals and head-on confrontations. But communication channels were always open.

Now they are closed — at least most of the time.

This experience has been a real test of our marriage. We consider ourselves fairly strong people and relatively well adjusted. We operate from the same theological base. We've thought out very clearly where we are through the years.

Now our life together is tough!

Prolonged illness is taking its toll on us both.

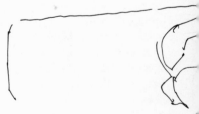

Sharp, unforgettable wipe-out
That blows all peace and sense of well-being
    from your mind.
It will surely be won, this uncontrollable tearing —
    ripping the end . . . just a piece of time.
Now I'm beginning to see what people mean
    when they speak of personal suffering.
It's down in your guts.

"But our sexual relationship has always been an important part of our marriage, and because its mutual enjoyment is gone, I now realize death has come to another area of human existence..."

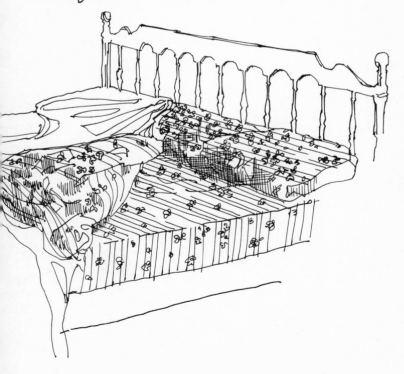

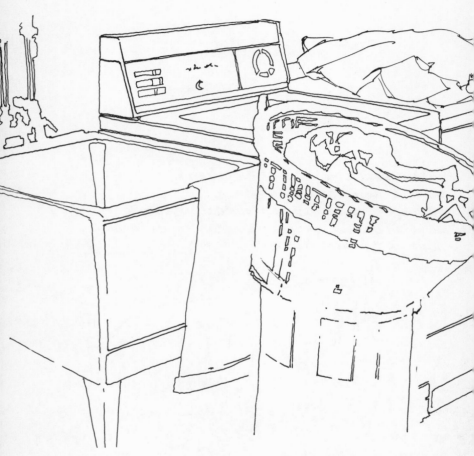

"... the little jobs I do
that affirm me as a worthwhile,
contributing person have
become my priorities."

I suppose the one great problem I confront which affects all of my emotional stability is the perspective of reality. And that affects my priorities.

I feel like part of my free fall is losing touch with reality. A less active person might react differently. But for an activist, maintaining a sense of reality becomes an awful test. It is hard to accept my limitations. I force myself to take naps. I force myself to be dependent.

The meaning of reality comes in the life I experience today — pills, pain, a small circle of friends, and in the satisfaction of doing the things I have always done. There is fulfillment in doing the laundry, in making a meal, in sewing Peanuts cartoons on work shirts for the children. And Gordon raises questions of priorities — the ones I should confront, but I can't. They have changed radically since the first months of my illness.

For example, my priorities should be in thinking through the meaning of changing ideas and values in this experience and recording it, in spending more time trying to get "into the heads" of our foster children, in establishing a better relationship with Gordon and working through with him a clearer understanding of my memorial service and the disposition of my body. But these concerns are not a part of my reality any more. They were at first, but in the intervening months the little jobs I do that affirm me as a worthwhile, contributing person have become my priorities.

I soon learned that the aura which surrounds a dying person created an irresistible desire to manipulate. Especially if you are a strong person, like I am, who has always been tempted to direct the lives of others.

The easiest thing in the world for me to do is take advantage of people who say, "Is there anything I can do?" by engineering a response to feed my ego needs. And no one in my family is going to make a big issue of something I want to do or buy, or the way I act because, "After all, we need to understand that Mother is dying. She is not her usual self, and so we ought to try and please her as much as possible."

Early in my illness I recognized this temptation. Because I am a strong person, used to controlling not just myself but others as well, this has been an enormous temptation I have seldom resisted.

Even from my sick bed I have tried, and usually succeeded, to control the operation of our home, including the discipline of our foster children. And this takes a lot of manipulation of feelings and a great deal of strength.

So when Brian announced in June of 1973 that he was going to

Jamaica, it about blew my mind. "I'm dying and you're taking a four-week trip to Jamaica?" I asked him. "I could be dead before you get back!" And there were tears to make him feel guilty.

But I'm married to a strong man, and we have strong children who aren't controlled easily. Their father supports them by telling them, "You must be your own person." And with great reluctance, I agree. Nevertheless, this is hard for all of them. "She's sick and therefore I can or can't do this" is one of the real issues they all confront daily.

As for me — it's still hard for most people to tell me, a dying person, "No!" That is, for most all — except my family!

There are times when I want to give up everything and surrender to Gordon and my family — "Do it the way you want." But then I find myself setting it up so that it can't happen.

My great desire to control has made it impossible for me to share the burden of our home with anyone else, although we need that help desperately. And that control mechanism has caused me to create a psychological strategy to assure me that after my death my children, husband, and friends will grieve and function according to my own wishes.

When I spoke to a group of chaplains about this, I was criticized strongly for manipulating my family through their grief. "That's not your right to do," one told me.

It's weird to think of controlling others' destinies after you're gone. And rationally I know it can't be done. But that doesn't stop me from trying.

For example, I have told groups that the memorial service will be marked by celebration, where there will be a band, music, laughter, and dancing. It will be a joyous experience in which we will celebrate the meaning of life and death — "WE," is what I said. I can't conceive of its happening any other way, and it will include ME. I've already programmed who will grieve the most and how they will show it. Now to the reader that will sound strange — but to those who know me it's understandable.

I will try to control until drugs or disease make that impossible.

And it is difficult for one who has always accepted and enjoyed responsibility to realize that as the disease progresses, others must make decisions for me. I have always been strong-willed — as has Gordon — and if there was any conflict in our relationship before my illness it centered in the question of control. Now I am losing it and with it my sense of destiny. Life for others will go on without me. And that adjustment is unbearable, for the control of my destiny and the reality of my own life are inextricably related. When I lose one, I lose the

82

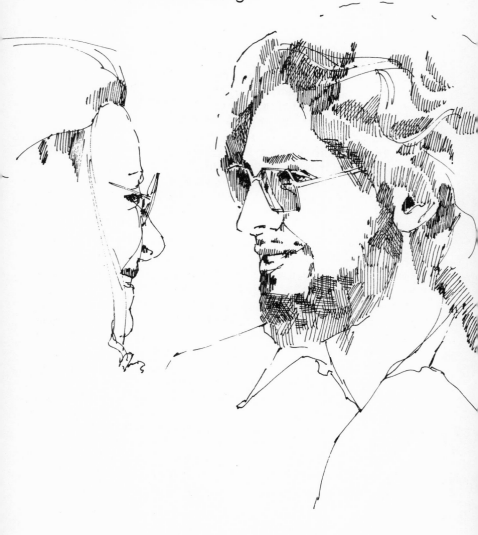

"... we have strong children
who aren't controlled easily."

other. That's why it is so hard for an independent person like me to die.

I believe Gordon fails to understand that the only way I can cope with my fear of what is happening is to remain independent. The more he tries to relate, the more fiercely independent I become. "You can only love me when I am dependent on you — when I am down or have my back to the wall — or in my sick bed asking for your help," I say to him. Somehow I can only communicate that need for independence through my hostility towards him and my rejection of him.

A prime example of this occurred one April evening in 1974 when we went to a Minnesota Symphony concert. He had angered me at dinner, so I told him I would go alone. He insisted on coming, but we were late and he let me off at the door so I could get in before the first number was performed. At its conclusion he joined me. My hostility was so great I tried to ignore him the whole evening.

When we left, he attempted to hold my arm so that I wouldn't fall down the steep steps of the auditorium. But I was soon way ahead of him and, though unsteady, made it down alone — almost lost in the crowd. Outside, I managed to keep one step ahead so he couldn't reach me. Finally he had taken all he could and, as before, leveled with me. "It's a great tragedy," he said, "that only when you fall on your face or when you are finally on your death bed will you realize that you are human and must depend on other persons."

Although I have never felt that Gordon really understands — or that anyone else does for that matter — I understand him — and I don't like it. I will survive without him!

But, then, why do I feel such a longing — such a need for others? And why don't people see me as someone who needs? As someone alone?

It doesn't take a psychiatrist to perceive the immense hostility that is deep within me. And now in a drawn-out terminal illness it often surfaces — and with bitterness. Not only because the life I love is being cut short, but because again I feel that I have failed — failed to complete the goals I set for myself — failed somehow to find the satisfaction and joy I know is out there, if I could only reach it. So when people ask, "What's bugging you anyway?" the only honest answer I can give is, "Me."

During the ten postoperative days in December, 1972, and January, 1973, I developed hypercalcemia, which means that the amount of calcium in the bloodstream was elevated to such a point that it affected my brain. I discovered later that during this hypercalcemic crisis I was close to coma, and if this had not been recognized

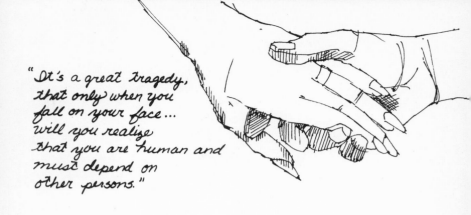

"It's a great tragedy, that only when you fall on your face ... will you realize that you are human and must depend on other persons."

and corrected I would have died. This condition caused me to hallucinate and to become very irrational — to such an extent that I had to be restrained. The hallucinations were frightening, and I still remember some of them very clearly.

They had a recurring theme which always found me trapped, either behind a wall or in a circumstance of my own making. My psychiatrist helped me interpret them as representing my struggle against the unmet goals and objectives I had established for myself. It was the replaying of a tape since childhood — my inability to measure up to the standards and goals I set for myself because of obstacles that seemed insurmountable. That created a trapped feeling that I cannot seem to escape. This, in large measure, accounts for the hostility I experience and the uncontrollable desire to make something out of my life even if it requires alienation from those for whom I care the most. These feelings are intensified by the knowledge that time is rapidly running out and I still haven't done all I want to do.

Even before I was sick the motivation to reach my goal — whether it was to open up the traditional church so that women and young people would have equal leadership opportunities or to prove that blacks and whites could live together in peace — gave people the impression that I was a rebel and irresponsible, besides.

My outspoken frankness and open hostility with those who disagreed caused me to be labeled a "hippie" in the annual church meeting when I aligned myself with the youth. And when we moved to the edge of the ghetto, surrounded by blacks, with blacks in our home, many thought we had lost our minds, but my motivation was to prove to myself that I could do what some said was impossible.

I treasure a poem written by my son when he was seventeen. It was lettered by a friend and is framed on the mantle of the fireplace in our bedroom:

To my Mother,

Look through the clearing smoke of conflicts
Through the dismal clouds of dismay.
You'll see her kneeling quite serenely
As she bows her head to pray.

For hers is the God of revolution,
Peaceful but radical nevertheless.
For people are different; ideas are varied
And everyone has their own to express.

Love
Brian

While I feel trapped by my limited life, I also feel a sense of freedom which comes in knowing that because life will soon be over, the restraints and inhibitions of our culture's value system become unimportant.

Perhaps the best illustration of this is my freed-up life-style which permits me to do what I feel rather than what seems to be "proper" and suitable.

For example, I do a lot of hugging and kissing of people I don't even know. If you feel free to love — why not?

One Sunday we took all of the young people in our house to our favorite black church, where the pastor is a good friend of ours. It was a great 2½-hour experience. When you consider that eight restless teenagers who went with us sat that long in church, that's got to be a real experience.

Because we have had blacks living in our home, I know that a show of affection between white women and black men isn't accepted exactly with enthusiasm by either race. And so when we got up to have this "be friends with each other" type thing in the service, I thought, "Well, I'll just be friends with everybody!" So I hugged and kissed the black men and tickled the toes of the babies. I'm sure that some white women would have been in shock. But the people there all seemed to like it. I've never been shy and retiring, but now I feel really free — what have I got to lose!

Unfortunately that freeing experience has also created some negatives in terms of relationships with others.

As my illness progresses, I experience alienation from those who have been close to me, and because of their proximity they are easy targets for my hostility. This has become of some concern to me. Strange it isn't more. I've always been a caring person, but now I really don't think reconciliation is that important. That troubles me, at times, but I rationalize it by telling myself that my time is so limited and my emotional strength so weak — it's not worth the effort. I no longer feel constrained to try. And that only increases my sense of aloneness.

These feelings of separation and loneliness have caused much of my depression.

When my friend John Sundquist left for a trip to Detroit, even though he would be back in two weeks, I felt it was our final good-bye. And I think he asked himself, "Will she be alive when I come back?" It's an unsettling, uncertain way to live. And it is a very awful, lonely, separating feeling. Nobody can change that for me.

Someone said the way we handle the many separations which come in our life's experiences will determine how we face the biggest one — death. And I have always found all separation very hard.

There are two facets to my sense of separation — closely related, but different.

The first is that feeling of aloneness. That is being all alone because no one else can be with you no matter how much you want him or how much he wants to be with you. It is the feeling of the free fall. You must do it alone.

But there is also loneliness in separation.

Loneliness is a sense of emptiness — caught without a way out.

Loneliness is being abandoned.

Loneliness is without company.

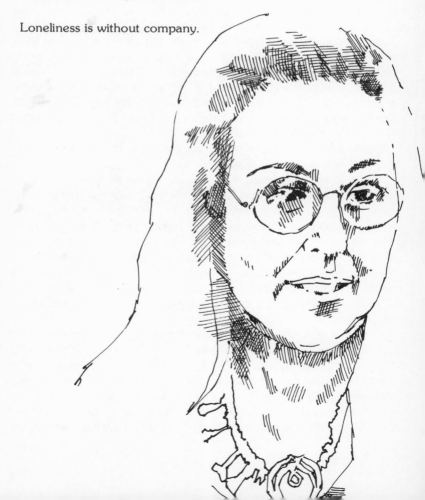

Job has provided the Christian apologist with the classic example of the one who suffers and who tries to find an answer for his scourge. In that beautiful Old Testament poetry we find portrayed his utter sense of loneliness and of abandonment.

> Know then that God has put me in the wrong,
> and closed his net about me.
> Behold, I cry out, "Violence!" but I am not answered;
> I call aloud, but there is no justice.
> He has walled up my way, so that I cannot pass,
> and he has set darkness upon my paths.
> He has stripped from me my glory,
> and taken the crown from my head.
> He breaks me down on every side, and I am gone,
> and my hope has he pulled up like a tree.
> He has kindled his wrath against me,
> and counts me as his adversary.
> His troops come on together;
> they have cast up siegeworks against me,
> and encamp round about my tent.
> He has put my brethren far from me,
> and my acquaintances are wholly estranged from me.
> My kinsfolk and my close friends have failed me;
> the guests in my house have forgotten me;
> my maidservants count me as a stranger;
> I have become an alien in their eyes (Job 19:6-15).

I can identify—

—with his feelings of alienation from his family and friends

—with his need for understanding and human empathy

—with his craving for God's presence, relationships, and an understanding of his fate.

I need to know that God has not abandoned me, but accepts me with all my human weakness, my questions, my fears, my doubts, my ambivalence, and my contradictions.

I need the affirmation of my humanity that Rita gave me when she entered my hospital room and through my tears assured me, "Don't be afraid — don't feel bad about crying — our Lord didn't want to die and he cried the night through. Even on the cross he felt the loneliness and the separation — just try to be a person — don't try to be an angel."

And I hear others ask, "Why should you feel that you can escape that same sense of aloneness, desperation, and fear?" I hear them trying to assure me that just because I am a Christian, I will not escape the emotions I am experiencing. I hear John Burns and Wayne assure me that no matter what the pain and drugs do to me, people will not remember that, for they know that is not the real JoAnn. They will remember me as I was before cancer transformed me into what I now am.

But the rationale and the logic are lost in my emotions.

"I believe; help my unbelief" (Mark 9:24).

I have come to believe that the defense mechanisms we use aren't as bad as I have always thought they were. In the era of sensitivity and T-groups, I believed and practiced openness of one's personal feelings. Even when such groups almost destroyed some strong people I knew, I felt there was a value in groups stripping away people's defenses so they could be known for what they were.

Now I'm sure I was wrong — for my defenses are strong, and without them I cannot cope. Therefore, it is becoming increasingly difficult for me to open up and be honest in expressing my feelings to others.

For example, in the months which followed my December, 1972, hospitalization, I would become extremely depressed — especially at the prospect of my next treatment. Almost like clockwork the two days before my treatment (scheduled every other week), I struggled with the question of whether or not I should permit my physician to treat me. He and I had long and serious discussions about it.

I'm not sure how honest I really was in trying to keep the issue on a moral or ethical level. It's true I have some intellectual problems with an act which assures certain death. But is it suicide to refuse that which will prolong your life? I believe strongly that an overdose of sleeping pills is wrong. And I often considered that route and discussed it with Gordon, my physicians, and friends. Their answers were almost unanimous, "That's your decision to make." And somehow I felt they were not only sympathetic with how I felt, but in similar circumstances would have taken that "out" for themselves.

Stewart Alsop said that terminal patients should be allowed to choose death through an active act of euthanasia.

Euthanasia doesn't sound too bad to someone in my situation. It comes from the Greek word meaning "a good or peaceful death." It can come either passively or actively. The former allows the physician to withdraw life-supporting machines or medication. My covenant with Wayne and John is that they will practice this form of euthanasia when the time comes. Most physicians surveyed find little problem with this.

To practice it actively is to administer medication that may relieve pain but hasten death.[1] One close friend volunteered to administer an overdose of morphine when and if I wanted it. He said a physician could not do that because of his Hippocratic oath, but he was not so bound and could do it for me.

I began to hoard sleeping pills so I had enough if, in fact, I decided on this way out. But I always stopped short before taking that kind of drastic action. I asked Wayne what would happen if I failed. The stomach pump and more hospitalization were great deterrents — almost as much as the moral question of whether or not it was right to take my own life.

For me, suicide is a sin — one I'm sure God forgives in similar situations — but somehow I don't want my life to end on that note. It would deny the strength of my faith. It would hurt my family. But most of all, I still have that overwhelming fear of death. And suicide is death. I would be just as dead as I will be when the normal course of my disease is completed. I don't want to die then. I don't want to die now.

And I guess that's basically why I can't stop treatments. In the final analysis it has little to do with anything except my fierce desire to live.

Early in my illness I tried to find some way out of the dilemma of using drugs to cover my pain.

My mother told me, "If I had to do it over again, I would never have had the surgery. I would have let cancer take its course as quickly as possible. It's been so hard on Daddy." She was referring to her abnormal, irrational behavior (caused by drugs) which created such anxiety for my dad. As a railroad engineer, he would be gone fifteen hours at a time and never knew what to expect when he came home. Once he returned to find the kitchen gas stove on but without a flame. He feared that in desperation and under the influence of drugs, she might try to take her life. But that was totally inconsistent with her normal responsible behavior. She was a valid Christian, totally confident, with a faith I felt was far stronger than mine.

But she had become a totally different person to me. She wasn't the mother I knew and remembered. She was a person under the heavy influence of drugs.

And I didn't want that to happen to me.

The use of drugs creates another conflict with my faith stance. I know that Jesus refused drugs offered him on the cross. Therefore, shouldn't I?

I became convinced, intellectually, that if someone else could enter the experience with me they could share my pain, even to the end.

---

[1] *Last Rights,* by Marya Mannes, published by William Morrow, is an excellent treatise on this subject.

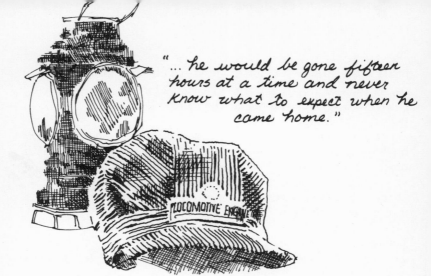

"... he would be gone fifteen hours at a time and never know what to expect when he came home."

That's one reason physical relationships have become so very important to me. The touch of another person is very helpful to me because I believe my pain can be shared. It's something akin to natural childbirth — a discipline of self-hypnosis. Then drugs would not be needed. I still believe that. But no one in my circle of close friends is mystical enough to achieve this — or, if so, has the ability to pull it off.

When I accepted this sharing as unrealistic in my own experience, I asked Wayne to keep my drugs at a low level even to the end so that I could remain clear and lucid.

Wayne and I agreed to a slow buildup of medication in response to pain, knowing that it would lead to dependence on chemicals to make life bearable.

I rationalize the morality of drug use by recognizing that I can't function as a person unless I can find relief from both pain and depression. But I discovered that the cycle created by drug use was impossible to break. The morphine creates depression. And the depression reduces my pain level, creating the need for more morphine.

Slowly, but surely, drugs are taking their toll on my personality and my ability to function rationally.

First, there were the intravenous treatments, Cooper's regimen, which succeeded in containing the tumor activity for twelve months. Then I was treated with a relatively new drug, Adriamicin, an antibiotic first manufactured in Italy and discovered to be successful in the treatment of cancer tumors.

Wayne requisitioned it from the National Cancer Institute, but after six months those treatments were stopped. The side effects beyond that point proved to be more dangerous than the disease. At that point

92

Wayne felt we had a partial remission. In July, 1974, Wayne started me on halotestin, a male hormone used to retard the growth of tumors caused by breast cancer. We hoped this would maintain my remission.

The chemotherapy drugs administered intravenously were supplemented orally with morphine for pain, Dalmane for sleep, Elavil for depression, Atarax as a booster for the morphine and cortisone derivatives like prednisone. The latter causes my body to retain liquids and gives a bloated effect. For that I take diuretics. I take twenty-six pills daily, more or less.

Small wonder that I find myself increasingly forgetting, so that I try to write as much down as I can. The frustration of being sure I did something only to find it undone often leads to emotional outbursts which remain unaccounted for in the family.

After eighteen months I find the morality of drug use as unresolved as when I first confronted the probability of addiction in my own life. Now I am content to let that moral problem be solved by the profession that has created it — medicine. Religion brings insight to resolving it, but since medicine must bear the consequence of its practice, it must solve it. As the ethical theologian can help to determine the nature of life, only medical science can determine when it is ended. The dialogue between medicine and ethics continues in an effort to determine at which point life is ended and when the plug should be pulled from the device which keeps a body functioning.

In the use of drugs the moral issue to be faced is, in my opinion: At what point do drugs destroy the quality of life and so alter one's personality that his ability to function as a person ceases? When does "better living through chemistry" reverse itself to destroy the quality of life?

Along with these questions I have asked myself, "What is the alternative?" The only alternative is suffering. Even though drugs have altered my personality, I do not feel that I, or others, should have to suffer. "I never take even an aspirin — for a toothache or a headache," a former drug addict told me. He had been through the terror of chemical dependency and was never again going to allow any semblance of it in his body.

But for me, chemical dependence is now the only way I can exist.

At the end of an address I made before a Lutheran congregation, a young man with two small children approached me with a question he had already raised with Gordon. The question was, "You say you have asked your doctors not to use heroic methods to keep you alive artificially, not to keep your body functioning by machine — what is the prolongation of life through chemicals?"

Gordon had given his answer. Now it was my turn.

Without knowing what Gordon had said, I admitted that this was a brand-new thought for me and I would need to think it through much more thoroughly, but my immediate response was, "At least this way I can still function as a person." And then I discovered Gordon had said the same thing.

Now I have thought about this more. I have tried to determine what it means to be a person. I'm not the same as I was eighteen months ago — or two years ago — or ten years ago when I was in good health. My personhood has deteriorated. My ability to function rationally as a constructive and contributing member of society, as a mother to our extended family, as a demonstrative wife to my husband, and as an independent person has been waning rapidly.

Since my illness, my personal experiences have demonstrated a decreasing quality of life. I have come to the point where I have serious moral questions as to how much longer I should be allowed to exist without the ability to enjoy the emotions, the reasoning process, and the personality that once created a quality of life that was positive, that was shared with others to make their lives better, and that was, for me, uncomparably rich.

The reality of where we are going with prolonged illness has turned into an eighteen-month nightmare for most of the time. A contemporary playwright said, "Humankind cannot bear very much reality."

To say that as a Christian I have found the spiritual strength to face the emotional problems of my illness is a cop-out — it's denial at its worst. One's personal relationship with God and the reality of Christ's presence do not eliminate the very human desire to control, or the angry hostility and depression I feel. These feelings haven't been removed simply because my basic commitment is to a Christian life-style. But that life-style can help me to deal with these emotional conflicts creatively.

Instead of staying in bed with my face toward the wall waiting to die, as many cancer patients do, or instead of spending hours crying hysterically because of a fear which has possessed me, I can cope with my crisis creatively. I have not escaped the hysterics or the depression. But I have learned to accept them as the human feelings that come because God has created me that way. And in that belief I cannot be utterly destroyed by what is happening to me.

Although I am alone most of the time in working through these emotions, I know there are many willing to work them through with me. They accept me regardless of my moods and encourage me to say, "I hate," when I do and, "I love," when I do. To me, that is

94

creative. At least my emotions are not buried, where they can grow and ultimately destroy me as surely as the growth of my tumor will.

I have tried to share with those willing to learn that the dying person handles these emotional conflicts in a variety of ways. At least I have.

The main character in *The Pawnbroker* states the desperate feeling I so often have. "I couldn't do anything. I couldn't do anything," he said. So I manufacture great new denial mechanisms and psychological walls to keep me from the knowledge that there is nothing I can do.

I have used a variety of these coping mechanisms in these long months. After the first operation I lived with the hope that since it was a clean job, everything would be OK. The second time I was not so sure — there was less hope. And the third time I was absolutely sure there was no hope. Then hostility became the mechanism by which I coped with most of the crises I experienced from then on, until I discovered a new dimension in hope.

That hope came in a rediscovery of purpose for my life. In that discovery I found the truth that Grandfather tried to teach me through what I thought was a very strange story. He came to my hospital room in late December of 1972 to say good-bye before he had to return to Omaha. We both thought we would never see each other again, and he wanted to leave me some word of hope.

He told me of an incident recorded in Judges 14:5-9 when young Samson came to the vineyards of Timnah and was attacked by a young lion. The Bible says that with his bare hands Samson "tore the lion asunder as one tears a kid."

He left the carcass, but a few days later returned to find in the body of the lion a swarm of bees and their honey. Samson scooped up the honey, brought it to his parents, and they all shared the taste of its sweetness.

"My prayer," Grandfather said to me, "is that somehow you will find sweetness in the bitterness of your death experience."

Out of his long years of experience as a minister, he has developed a faith that even in the midst of suffering and death, good can come to those who believe.

Whatever "sweetness" I have tasted in these months, whatever good has come, has come because I found a new purpose for my life. My life is slowly being spent to help others to understand what is happening to me and to provide a home for those who need what I have to offer them. That purpose has given me a new sense of worth and a new kind of hope — that the lives of others will become more meaningful because of mine.

I don't have time to die — at least right now.

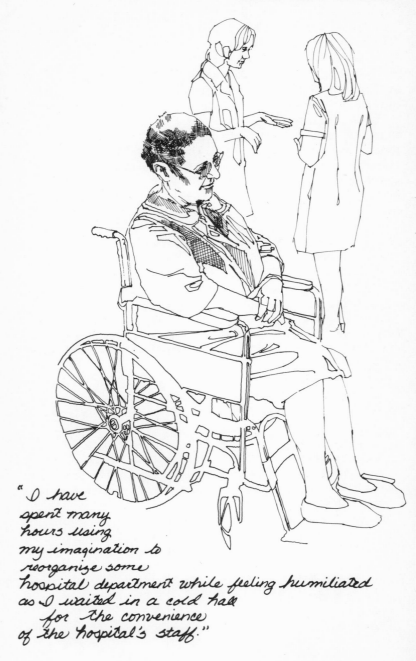

" I have
spent many
hours using
my imagination to
reorganize some
hospital department while feeling humiliated
as I waited in a cold hall
for the convenience
of the hospital's staff."

It's night now.
About the only way you can tell
   is by the procedures.
The little medical dances, done in precision,
   are the markings of getting well.
Undoubtedly these mechanisms,
   some a little more sophisticated,
Have been taught since the medical profession
   began to jell.
First, one must wash one's hands, one's teeth, and
   "use the facilities." That way you won't have to
   disturb a night nurse with something so simple as
   "I need the pan —" and feel very much like a naughty
   child.
How is it that such a little request — day or night —
   is of such great significance?
It is so important — sometimes important enough to
   measure and write carefully on a "news-sheet."
Sheet: now that is another very vital cog in the
   "getting well" syndrome.
Sheets AND their importance have a lot to do with the
   age of the nurse, the preparation AND experience.
Now this is not ALWAYS SO. Sometimes during all these years of
   learning nursing, a "touch rebel" arises. But by the
   time three years have passed, a good deal of that
   creativity has been consistently beaten out of the student.
   She has forgotten all about touch . . . .
We are hoping that by the third year, any student who
   amounts to much has carefully been taken care of
   and the "touch — feel" is gone. Any student who amounted
   to much could give total care without ever touching
   the patient either physically or emotionally. Patients
   are not there for personal encounter; they are there to
   get well.
The younger nurses seem to be catching on to this involvement.
   Hurrah!
To be an efficient nurse, they see to it that their patients
   are all taken care of in plenty of time so as not to
   disturb coffee break. They should have been technicians.
A dying patient needs a compassionate person who happens
   to be a nurse who cares about that patient as a single,
   needy person.

97

Deprofessionalizing the Physician

I have referred to all my doctors by their first name — nurses and ministers, too — because they are part of my support system, for one thing, and because I am committed to humanizing them. There's nothing more professional than the term "doctor." So mine are Wayne, Vince, John, and Jerry. That makes them persons, and that's how I want to relate to them.

That's the basis of my whole support system — to have people deal with me as a person, not as a patient or a responsibility. To provide that support for any patient requires more than many are willing to give because it means getting into the lives and heads of people. Perhaps that's why many in the helping professions must remain professional. They can't handle the requirements of a relationship that sees people as persons rather than responsibilities.

Among some physicians that professionalism is evidenced by viewing patients as a kind of job they've done. So they come into the patient's room with their entourage of nurses. If they happen to be surgeons, they rip the covers off and they examine their work to see whether or not they did a good job. I was very fortunate because I had a very sensitive surgeon who always asked me, "How's it going? Do you have any complaints?" Then he would look at his work. But this is not true of all surgeons.

That kind of professionalism makes it very hard to cope with dying patients because dealing with those patients requires a special sensitivity. I was told by one doctor that the most important factor in caring for a dying patient is candor. That affirms the patient as a person who has a right to know what is happening to him. It has never failed. The patient does not become more depressed by knowing what is wrong with him.

And he said the family reacts the same way. So nurses and physicians should provide leadership in dealing with dying in a direct way. But I suspect many will not admit to themselves the possibility their patient is going to die while under their care.

Denial of the death diagnosis often is as real to those who care for the patient as it is for the patient himself. And they do everything in their power to keep that patient alive.

I suppose one reason death is so difficult for members of the medical profession to confront is that it represents defeat. They have been taught to heal, or at least aid the healing process, and for the patient to die is to fail. No one wants to fail.

Death should be thought of as the logical end of existence, but it is more often viewed as a scientific enemy. We do everything we can to prevent it. If we can't, we have somehow failed.

But doctors haven't found all of the answers either, so they can't save everybody. When they have learned to accept that, perhaps they will learn to talk with patients honestly about their condition. "Well, JoAnn, you're failing. You're not quite as good today as you were yesterday," they could say. Or: "This disease progresses this way and this is what you can expect. When your body gets to a certain point, we can do no more."

I know that not all physicians can handle dying that way, and I realize that it doesn't necessarily follow that those who do well in curing and controlling disease will also do well in the care of the dying.

If the physician can't level with the family or with the patient for one reason or another, then he should try to discover if there is a clergyman or priest who can.

Successfully coping with what we interpret as failure is not unique to the medical profession.

Gordon and I have read books and attended lectures on how to handle your teenagers successfully. What you are rarely told is that sometimes you will fail. Then what? In our home we have had over forty teenagers whose home life has somehow failed them. We have talked to some of their parents, who in anguish and deep despair, wonder, "Where have we gone wrong?"

Somehow we have failed to learn to handle failure. Perhaps this is because our culture is so success-orientated that we deny failure as a real option. For the Christian, this denial has become part of a false theological structure which views failure as the result of being out of God's will.

Gordon and I have felt the need to understand what it means to fail whether it be at work, in relationships, or in our home. We have also felt the same anguish, guilt, and hurt experienced by the parents of some of our foster children when we, too, have failed in dealing with their problems.

Because the medical community views failure in the same way, it was not too surprising to hear Dr. Elisabeth Kübler-Ross tell of her early attempts to interview dying patients in a Chicago hospital, only to discover great reluctance at each nursing station to admit that there were dying or critically ill patients there. The hospital staff could not freely admit this failure. In one of my many hospital experiences I met one head nurse who was proud of her record of twenty years with no deaths while she was in charge. They died on the next shift.

The reality of death and the failure it represents must be confronted by the medical community more creatively and realistically.

Death education is too late in the hospital room when the verdict "terminal illness" is announced. From my personal experience such education was needed years ago and would have made these long months more livable. I'm not laying this responsibility totally on the medical profession, but I do believe that death education should be a part of the curriculum of every medical and nursing school so that the physician and the nurse can give leadership in helping the dying patient face the normal and ultimate in human experiences.

One of the reasons cited for the failure of the medical community to deal with terminal patients is they "can't deal with the anxieties and problems of their own deaths and, therefore, they avoid dealing with the anxieties and problems of their own patients," according to Robert L. Scheig, chief of gastroenterology at the University of Connecticut Medical School (in a May 1, 1974, news article in the *St. Paul Dispatch*).

If this problem were confronted early in their educational experience, they would be prepared to deal more effectively with the terminal patient.

In the same article, Edward F. Dobihal, Jr., director of the Department of Religious Ministries at Yale New Haven Hospital in Connecticut, says: "Health care workers receive gratification through healing, through giving. When they no longer can give, there is no gratification, so the terminal patient is avoided. Discussion with him is restricted for fear the topic of death will arise."

Humanizing the Hospital

Underlying many complaints of patients, whether they are dying or not, is the feeling that they are being treated as "nonpersons" while hospitalized. Justified or not, they believe there is a lack of sensitivity on the part of many professionals who work with sick people. This feeling is the result of a dehumanizing process which often takes place unconsciously in dealing with the sick.

It happens when doctors and nurses talk to the chart or at the patient rather than to him. It happens when hospital personnel fail to use the two-tenths of a second it takes to say good morning — and to call the person by his name, or to use a little more time to introduce themselves to the patient.

That would tend to alleviate the feeling I've often had that patients are viewed by some hospital people as robots — like they are in a cubicle — waiting to be serviced, serviced in such a way that in a few days they will be exchanged for some other patients.

But the fact of the matter is some of us won't get out — and we're the ones who need some extra "strokes," which require that the hospital personnel give more of their time and more of themselves. I appreciate the nurse or the aide who stops in often to see what I need, even if it's only assurance. There's nothing worse than to be left alone for forty to forty-five minutes with a friendly television set or radio to keep you company. To my way of thinking, there's nothing more impersonal than that intercom to which you speak your requests and which answers coldly, "I'll have someone come down in a minute."

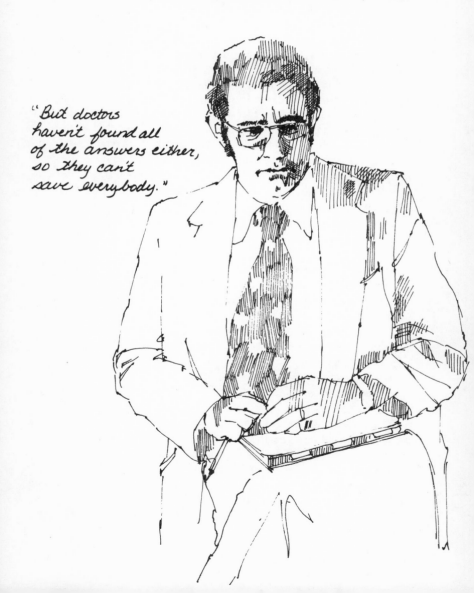

"But doctors haven't found all of the answers either, so they can't save everybody."

That can be completely demoralizing, like being totally isolated in a faraway place where nobody gives a rap about you.

Waiting on a cart for an X-ray procedure or in a chair for a lab test also becomes demoralizing to one who really feels sick. An occasional word of assurance from a technician or, better yet, an explanation of the time lag would make me feel like a person instead of a patient waiting to be processed.

I have spent many hours using my imagination to reorganize some hospital department while feeling humiliated as I waited in a cold hall for the convenience of the hospital's staff.

It is difficult for me to believe that a hospital employee sensitized to the feeling one has as a nonperson would ever allow that to happen to another patient.

In the movie *Hospital* there were two caricatures of hospital situations which come too close to the truth in portraying conditions in some big and busy hospital communities. In one situation the movie's "villain" was trying to lose a patient and finally decided to park his hospital cart in the hall of the X-ray department. That way, he said, the patient wouldn't be noticed for many hours, even days. In the other scene a coronary patient brought to the emergency room was pronounced dead after several hours of waiting. Cause of death — "neglect."

Dehumanizing also comes when my physician or nurse does not take time to explain what medication I am taking and why I am to take it.

For me, this has been a minimal problem in my hospitalization because I have steadfastly refused to take anything without an explanation. Nevertheless, I have the feeling a pain medication or a sleeping pill is administered to "keep the patient in 582 quiet so she will quit bugging us." And that's an awful feeling.

A few times I've had to tell the nurse "no" when she brought me medication with the word, "Your doctor wants you to have this." I have a right to accept or refuse it — whether or not it makes the nurse, or the physician, angry. Their responsibility is to tell me what it is and why I should take it.

Public pressure, the adoption of a patient's bill of rights by many hospitals, and the increasing sensitivity of the medical profession and hospital employees are making a marked change in the way we view patient's needs. But most of all, it must be the patient who insists on being treated as a person whose need is for wholeness, which never can come in the cold, sterile process of dehumanization.

My observation is that the private church-related hospital has been more responsive than public hospitals to the need for humanizing the whole healing process and of ministering to patients as persons. There are several reasons for this. One is that whether we like it or not health care is a competitive business. Therefore, to attract a good, active medical staff, private hospitals compete by trying to provide better facilities, service, and employees. Furthermore, the church-related hospital often attracts a staff motivated by service, rather than higher salaries and job security. Also, the private church-related hospital can shift gears more rapidly to keep pace with changing health-care trends. One of these is to make the hospital less sterile and more homelike. The result of these factors is usually a stronger emphasis on treating patients as persons. Often the smaller hospital can achieve this more easily than the larger ones.

From my own experience I have found that there *is* a difference between the larger public hospital and the smaller private ones.

Therefore, one of the most discouraging trends in the delivery of health care is increased government control and intervention.

Arguments for the justification of increased intervention are usually based on increased medical costs. But it is interesting to note that from January, 1971, through March of 1974, the Consumer Price Index for all costs rose 20 percent while medical care costs rose only 15 percent.[1] At the same time first-class mail costs increased 66 percent while 900 post offices were being closed and late afternoon pickups stopped in many communities. Also the discontinuation of Saturday and special delivery is contemplated in the near future. Second-class rates are scheduled to cost publishers of periodicals 242 percent more in 1976 than in 1971.[2]

I shudder to think what will happen to the private, church-related hospitals as government control increases. If that means the same kind of "personalized," "efficient," and "economical" service that we experience in our postal service, we are in for trouble.

If that happens, we can expect an intensification of an experience recorded by John Carmody. In an article titled "A Death, a Radicalization," he tells of the death experience of his sixty-year-old father:

Nurses and aides constantly putter about the dying patient, chatter at him, insist on "just another mouthful." They treat an intelligent 60-year-old like a preschooler, because he is moribund. Visitors are worse. They babble on and on — about

---

[1] Consumer Price Index published by the United States Department of Labor.

[2] From articles published in *Time,* vol. 103, no. 8, (February 25, 1974), p. 54; and *Dun's,* March, 1974 p. 67f.

the cards, the flowers, the food, the humidity. No one seems able to shut up, let alone contemplate, let alone pray. No, in that hospital death is a physiological problem and a cultural embarrassment. You have to be almost nasty if you would honor death's insistence on God's Lordship and Christ's cross. You have blatantly to contradict the hospital's whole style if death is to be a calm journey into the great unknown, a father's last lesson to his son.

The modern hospital is the greatest enemy of meaningful death. Thanatologists like Elisabeth Kübler-Ross *On Death and Dying* [Macmillan, 1970]) say that fear is the root of this hostility. Indeed, they find that fear of death is a significant motivation in those who enter medicine. I'd like to believe this analysis, because it helps me absolve my father's doctors. They did not visit him in his last days, and they have yet to communicate at all with us his family (except for their bill). My anger at them is beginning to turn into pity.[3]

My personal experience does not support Carmody's criticisms, but there is adequate evidence that his story, or parts of it, are duplicated far too often in the lives of too many people. That's why many private, church-related hospitals are doing all they can to humanize the healing process.

Carmody's experience does affirm a principle I have come to accept, namely, that environment is one of the most supportive factors in treating the sick and dying.

For example, a psychologist asked a group of hospital employees, "What is 'it' that heals in a hospital? Is 'it' the doctor, the patient, the nurse, the surgery, medicine?" He then suggested that healing takes place in an atmosphere in which persons can respond to the healing process. Whether they are terminally ill or not, they can be "healed" enough to be whole persons.

Someone suggests we should change the hospital environment from the traditional "Shhh—quiet" hospital zone to hello's, talk, laughter, and noise. Instead, signs should read, "Beware! Healing, too, can be contagious."

In an environment where there is smiling, conversing, sharing, and responding to the needs of others, the patient and those surrounding

---

[3] John Carmody, "A Death, a Radicalization," *The Christian Century* (vol. 91, no. 23), June 12-19, 1974, p. 639. Copyright 1974 Christian Century Foundation. Reprinted by permission.

him can continue to achieve personal growth as whole persons.

The development of that kind of atmosphere places a great deal of responsibility on the hospital staff, which often greets complaints with hostility and isolation. And that's understandable. But the patient who complains is on the way to recovery. A friend of mine said to a group of nurses: "Give that patient an eager response. Forget professional dignity. A complainer is an open person. Listen to his distress. Don't respond with 'nothing's wrong.' That's unreal, inhuman. Share your softness, your compassion." He called it "creative" complaining.

The angry, the hostile, the depressed dying patients require understanding if we are to deal with them effectively. To respond to an angry patient with anger never helps either the patient or the one who is responding. Because there is a failure to understand the underlying hostility and anger that many patients have, there is a failure to establish a healing relationship.

Any situation that increases depression or anxiety impedes healing. The mother who tells the frightened child, "Don't be afraid — everything's all right," doesn't make the dark go away or the ghosts in the closet disappear, but she conveys a trust in life, trust in being. And that allows for "everything will be all right."

That's what it means to humanize the support system needed by the sick and dying.

Environment has been one of the most supporting factors in my health care, being in familiar surroundings with familiar faces. In a totally strange environment I believe my recovery would be delayed in direct proportion to my ability to relate to where I was.

I remember, early in my illness, both John and Wayne feared I would follow the pattern of many cancer patients by just lying down and wasting away. For that reason they were always quick to get me home into my normal pattern of living and the familiar surroundings of my home. And I always agreed with that. I can remember one time during a long hospital stay when I wanted to be home so badly I would often imagine the smell of my dogs, whom I love and missed very much.

To push this to its logical conclusion — I hope to die at home, in my own bed, surrounded by my own family and the things which represent a large part of my emotional security. I personally believe that will be better for me than all of the skilled care and cleanliness of any hospital — no matter how good it happens to be.

This need has been taken into consideration in plans to build a $2.7 million facility in Branford, Connecticut, to provide for dying patients and their families. The facility will have forty-four beds and a round-

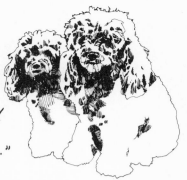

"... I wanted to be home so badly I would often imagine the smell of my dogs..."

the-clock home care service center to aid the majority of patients who are expected to prefer dying at home.

One of my strongest feelings about the hospital environment is that there should be two or three rooms equipped with double beds for conjugal visits. How often I wanted Gordon near me during the night and there were no medical reasons that prevented this. I believe it should be possible for a husband or a wife to stay with his or her mate, even if it is just overnight and if the patient doesn't need a lot of nursing care, particularly if it's a terminal disease and it's going to be a long hospitalization. That means night after night after night of going to sleep alone and having your fears and anxieties to face alone with nobody to talk with on the same level that you experience with your mate.

If your husband or wife could stay with you overnight, the healthy mate could take away a lot of the anxiety and even some of the pain by giving assurances that, "I will be here; I will support you; no matter what happens, you can count on me; we're in this together and I love you." That occurs in the nonverbal communication of simply sleeping together.

And I am fully convinced that a number of patients could go home, maybe days earlier, if they could have that kind of loving support from their mates.

By entering into a full physical relationship with you, staying by you all night, sitting by your bed, or placing their body near your body, they say, "I would like to share the pain with you."

Although the pain may not leave the sick person's body, I honestly believe that this is so supportive that it will have a healing effect.

A nurse asked me how I would like the hospital staff to respond. Would I like to have them come in, sit, and listen? My answer to that question always has been, "Yes." And I would like them to express their care and to tell me I'm an acceptable person — in other words give me some psychological "strokes."

But if they can't, at least they can hold my hand and say, "That was a bad blow," or "Today has been tough, hasn't it?"

Then I would know they care.

And if I cry, allow me to do that — and if they are really great people, they might cry with me.

But I could not initiate that contact. After all, I am not there to serve the nurse — but she is to serve me. One of my biggest criticisms of nurses is that they often treat the patient to fit into their pattern. Your nurse thinks, "I've got four patients to bathe before my coffee break." The feeling she communicates is, "You're going to brush your teeth now whether you like it or not." That creates great resistance in me because I hate to give up the priority of my being. I will determine that for myself. And I'll peel my own orange until I get so weak it keeps falling to the floor.

I realize the work pressure is often very heavy for a nurse — especially if occupancy is high and the station is short-staffed. But to be left alone when your anxiety is high or to be forced into a mold for the convenience of the hospital staff is dehumanizing and depressing.

I have come to believe that the ability to work effectively with patients is a gift which God has given to some nurses. It's a feeling that others can't acquire whether they are graduates of a junior college, diploma school, or a four-year college. I know some advanced-degree nurses whose bedside manner is intolerable — but I have also known some L.P.N.'s and aides who can relate to me in an extremely helpful way.

Grace is one of these gifted nurses. She would come to me in my darkest hours, do all that she could to make me comfortable — and just be there. And she came into my room often.

I remember one morning when she entered my room after a night of excruciating pain which the doctors were still unable to diagnose. I was afraid and hurting. She leaned down and whispered in my ear, "Do you want me to pray this morning?" I affirmed this need — and she did. Her prayer was brief, realistic, and supportive.

On another occasion she and a friend visited me after working hours just to see how I was doing. I was in good spirits that night so they asked if they could get me something to eat. "What would taste good?" Grace asked. "Pepperoni pizza," I said. And in less than an hour they returned with the best pizza I had ever eaten.

Grace has that gift of tuning in to where I am and responding to the need of that moment.

My dad was a railroad man for forty-five years — a "hoghead" that is, a freight engineer. He often used some crude but very explicit phrases. In the old days when he rode the coal-fired engines, he would say about some young apprentice crew member, "He'll never make it as an engineer — he doesn't have it in his butt." He knew that if the young man didn't have a certain "feel" for driving that engine he would never succeed. Some had it. Some didn't.

There are some who are born with the potential to develop into skilled nurses, who instinctively know when to act and interact with the patient — to encourage the healing process of the whole person. Others will never be more than technicians mechanically performing their duties, never learning to sensitize themselves to the feelings of those for whom they are to care.

Another example of what I mean is found in "Mum."

Mum, Gordon's mother, who came to stay with me in the winter of 1973, had a unique way of finding a balance between encouraging me and babying me. And she had no training as a nurse or any kind of health professional. She, too, is a strong woman. She is outspoken and has an indomitable will. So you would think we would clash constantly.

But Mum never helped me to my room unless I asked. After I returned home from the hospital that winter, I would often crawl up the stairs on my hands and knees because I was too unsteady to walk. She never offered to help but stood by watching so that I would not slip. She knew that the most important thing for me was to do it myself, not to be babied or humiliated by a helping hand that only reminded me of my inadequacy. She knew that if I needed help I would ask for it.

She treated me that way and slowly encouraged me to eat until my strength had been regained and I could function as a person again.

I guess the most humiliating thing a nurse ever did to me was in preparing me for discharge after one of my many hospitalizations. I had my big winter coat on and I was very hot, weak, and uncomfortable. All I wanted to do was get in that car and get home. I had had it for that day.

Then she said to me, "Oh, my dear — your hair is mussed, let's brush it out a little bit." She brushed my hair in a long curl like I was four years old. At the time I felt that was the greatest insult I'd ever had in my life. What difference did it make if my hair was messy? To put my hair in a little curl made me a dependent child. But I'm a forty-nine-year-old woman who wants to control her own life!

She was responding to her need to function as she was programmed without taking time to tune in to where I was or what I wanted as a person. She fulfilled a responsibility she saw as her duty — and left me a humiliated person.

And again I lost control.

I have noticed a distinct difference in nurses who are younger. They seem to be a product of a more sensitive education which teaches them the importance of human relationships and the dynamics of encounters with other human beings.

Younger nurses seem to be concerned about touch and feel, and feelings — getting into people's lives and caring about them as persons. They aren't all tied up with the old rules and regulations that stifle the effectiveness of nursing the patient to wholeness again. Those false rules inhibit the nurse so that she touches you very nimbly even to get a band-aid on. If the nurse is making the bed for a male patient, she is to be very careful to avoid his genital area. This might mean trouble! Nurses never sit on the bed — that's a very important rule, created by our sexual hang-ups, which has nothing to do with developing a helpful relationship in the healing process of that patient.

From a patient's point of view, there is a great advantage in having one nurse assigned to care for you. That nurse would soon come to know your moods, your symptoms, your emotional as well as physical needs, and, in time, could learn to minister in a supportive role. Through such a relationship just being there could do wonders in the humanizing of a helping profession and could speed the emotional healing of most traumatic physical problems.

Most nurses work from two assumptions: (1) the patient can be made comfortable and well again, and (2) the doctor and she know what is best for the patient.

The nurse who believes that rarely gets in touch with where I am in terms of my feelings, especially my hostility and anger. She is the one who enters the room early in the morning, throws open the curtains, and says, "Aren't we having a beautiful day?" or "Breakfast is coming. Wouldn't you like to brush your teeth now?" and "Won't we feel a lot better for breakfast if we wake up, enjoy the sun, and wash up!"

That's the worst thing a nurse can say to me when my anger is running high and resentment for my fate is in control. Although my doctors and nurses are often frustrated by their inability to relate to me because everything they seem to do is wrong, they can always count on my consistent response under such circumstances. My answer will be, "NO!"

When I am down emotionally, the first one to enter my room and turn the light on is in trouble — including the doctor. It raises all my antagonism.

The "we" and "our" make me feel like a child — and as though I have lost control. But I have the right to be treated as a person. That's part of the control of my own destiny, and that's what maintains my personhood.

109

I don't want someone else to assume control of my life until I can't do a thing about it.

That's something I resent more than anything else, whether it's caused by nurses, physicians, or my family.

I have been fortunate in having some nurses who reject these assumptions. They support me with expressions such as, "I'm really sorry you're going through this." They stop in often just to talk or to ask me what I need to be more comfortable. They ask me if I want breakfast and if I say, "No," they say, "OK," and let me decide when I'll get ready for it that morning.

I don't feel I should be cajoled to eat my meals, bathe, or take medication. Given the proper emotional climate and an understanding of the situation, I will do that on my own.

A nurse who is sensitized to people has a better idea of how to react to a patient who is resentful and angry. Operating on the principle of getting into my life, she comes in quietly in the morning and gets as close to me as possible, touches me gently, and asks, "JoAnn, how did you get along last night?" Then, if she waits a few minutes, I'll give her my agenda and we can get in touch with each other's feelings. I will tell her when or if I want breakfast and whether or not I'm able to take my own bath or shower.

But this is really an establishment problem that is solved in a more relaxed atmosphere where (1) the hospital's program is radically changed to accommodate the patient and (2) the entire staff is continually taught that the patient's needs are the most important. Then feeding the patients at a certain hour and bathing them by a predetermined time become secondary to the concern for the patient as a person. My experience is that the smaller, church-related private hospitals like Midway, where I have spent most of my hospitalizations, are moving rapidly in this direction.

Now I'm not suggesting that the whole dietary department should adjust their schedule for me. I realize the tray must be delivered to my room by a certain time, but I don't have to eat what's on it then.

There is a trend in many hospitals to prepare meals at the nursing station by using the same methods fast food chains have found both profitable and convenient. Frozen foods and microwave ovens installed on the stations would then permit patients to eat on their own schedule from a widely selected menu. That would go a long way towards humanizing service to patients.

And if I decided I didn't want a bath that particular morning, I'm sure that would not be a disaster. I bathe one-half as much at home, and in the hospital I suppose I have one-tenth less of a chance to get myself

110

dirty enough for a bath.

There is also a need to deprofessionalize and humanize the clergy in their relationships to the sick.

Deprofessionalizing the Clergy

One of my favorite targets in speeches I have given are pastors and students in clinical training for the chaplaincy. I often paint the caricature of one who has six patients to see, and only so much time in which to do it.

The usual ritual is to step to the end of the patient's bed and say, "Good morning, it's a nice day," or, if it isn't, some similar inane remark. But they avoid asking if the patient had a good or bad night because the answer might take too long.

Then the question always comes, "Would you like for me to read some favorite Scripture?" And I wonder, "Whose favorite?" It's not mine because he didn't take time to find out. But the "favorite" Scripture is always the same — it's amazing the insight they have!

Then, "Would you like me to pray?" That's always distressed me because I think, "How in the world do you know what to pray for on my behalf? You haven't even found out what my needs are."

A patient will tell a chaplain, his pastor, or a spiritual advisor where he is hurting and what his needs are if the visitor will exercise some degree of patience.

I would have told the many who visited me what my favorite Scripture is — if I had ever been asked.

I had one chaplaincy student visit me often. He was very handsome and obviously concerned about his appearance — more than his ability to relate. I really believe his preparation for entering my room was to comb his hair, straighten his tie, and make sure he looked his best. I honestly can't remember a thing he said to me during our many visits. He seemed paralyzed by his frequent contacts with me. I was really sick and wanted to talk about it. But all he felt required to do was call on me and help me "pass the time of day." Therefore, his talk was always inane.

All he needed to do was to be my friend, hold my hand, offer me a paper tissue if I cried — cry himself. Anything to get in touch.

To have someone cry with me is the most affirming experience I know. It says, "I know you must feel bad — and because I care about you, I feel bad, too." And if a person stays with me, eventually he will find the clue that can help him deal with some of the deepest needs I am only going to express to another human who can show me that he, too, feels. I know I can trust that person. And he *will* be able to help.

I've told pastors, "If you haven't time to develop a relationship like that with your parishioner, it's better to stay in the office and open the mail." At the same time I've told their parishioners, "You clowns should get out and do a little of this visiting and let your pastor do some other things. He has only so much time to visit the sick and dying and often just can't get into the lives of some of the people you can."

When *anyone* comes to visit me, I don't want him to come with his own agenda. This is a problem for anyone ministering to the sick. I often get the feeling that before people enter my room, they try to decide what to say. I don't want to hear their concerns. I want them to empty their heads of their own ideas. When you visit a sick person, fill your head with thoughts about that person, your care for him, and what you can do to get in touch with him.

For example, if your friend has had a stroke and has become very unattractive, simply get very close to him, hold his hand — assure him in every way that his appearance doesn't matter — and just wait. If he cries, give him a handkerchief and cry with him. Don't worry about what you're going to do — just be. Tell him, "I love you. I'll be there."

A Catholic Sister in the clinical pastoral education program at Midway Hospital came to see me very discouraged by her constant vigil at the side of a patient dying of cancer. She was waiting for the opportunity to get in touch — for that patient to open up and talk about her condition. But the patient wouldn't do that.

We talked about that often and agreed that the patient was denying her condition. It was the only way she could cope. I told the Sister, "Don't give up. Just keep on going."

If a dying person needs to play that game of denial, you needn't play it with him, but neither should you yank the support out. That's what I mean by getting in touch with where the patient is.

I know a couple who shared the same experience of prolonged illness that Gordon and I are having. They rarely spoke to their closest friends about it. And I doubt if they talked to each other very much about death. Denial was the only way they could cope with their crisis.

A few weeks before the husband died, I called the wife and simply said I had followed their case, was thinking of them, and knew how they were feeling. I said, "You needn't respond — I just want you to know I'm with you."

It was like turning the faucet on. She talked all about it. We didn't know each other well, but we identified. We were in the same situation and therefore were on the same wave length.

Another illustration of what I mean is found in the contrasting

112

reactions of two friends who came to see me after my first mastectomy. "You are a lucky girl," one said. He meant it sincerely. He meant that the tumor was found in time and apparently removed successfully. But he didn't know how I felt, and my response was, "You know how lucky I feel — it would be how you would feel if you had just been castrated." He made me feel the same way an eighteen-year-old nurse did, one who had never been sick a day in her life and who came in and said, "Keep looking up." A dying person doesn't need inane statements like that.

The other friend sat on my bed two days later and said, "You got a rotten deal — it's a damn shame." And I broke down. We were on the same wave length and a supportive relationship developed that really helped me.

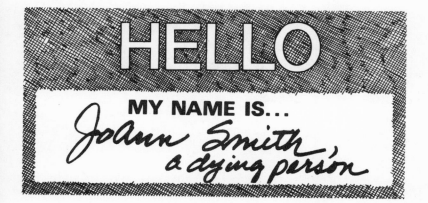

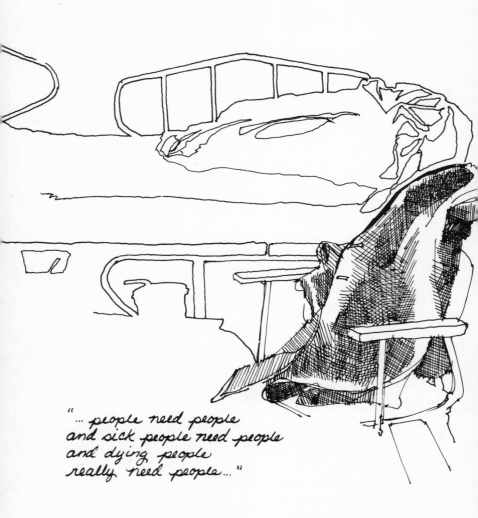

"... people need people
and sick people need people
and dying people
really need people ..."

I have very strong feelings about the fact that people need people and that sick people need people and that dying people *really* need people — because they need a support system. The only support system — it can't be done by a radio or a console — can be provided by other persons. A person who touches you, cares about you, listens to you, talks to you, helps you make the grade, pass the test, hold on, stand fast!

Sick people, especially most dying people, are very unpleasant to be around and so we avoid visiting them. I know because I was one who always avoided seeing them if I possibly could. I always rationalized to myself, "Well, I wouldn't know what to say."

But you don't need to say anything. If you just go in and listen, they'll do all the "saying" because they really want to talk about themselves. And they need to talk about themselves. They need to get in touch with their feelings and they need to tell it to another human. They may just want to tell you, "I'm really sick."

Or they may just want to remain silent. On one occasion my very close friends, Ray and Gladys, came to see me when I was deeply depressed. I cried through the whole hour of their visit. They didn't say a word but simply held my hand until they had to go.

By their action they simply affirmed me as a good person and assured me that I need not be ashamed of my depression or tears.

But don't sit there and say, "Oh, I'm sure you're getting better." You deny them the right of dealing realistically with their condition. They're sick and they know they're sick — or they're dying. And they know when they're dying! So don't tell them that they're not. Affirm them. Say, "I know it must be really difficult." If in good faith you can say, "You've really been a terrific person and I really care about you and I'm really going to miss you," that will help the person think, "My life has really been worthwhile. I've counted at least for one person."

When my friend Barbara was with me following the liver scan, she said, "You know, I've never been sick; what can I do for you?" And I said, "You just be Barbara." And she has responded that way. If I need to talk, she listens. And if I cry, she cries.

There is no need to feel we should hide our feelings from people who are dying — who want you to affirm the fact that they are dying. Don't lose control but don't hold back the tears in the presence of a dying patient. Grief is not a selfish emotion, and the dying cry for many people.

There are many who feel helpless in offering me support, and I remember that in my mother's dying experience, I felt as helpless as many feel in relating to me. Her deep faith in God made it appropriate for me to read Scripture and to pray with her often. Aside from that and washing her body, there was little else I could do but just be.

A great deal of the time that's what I want people to do for me. Just to be. And to relate to me as they always have.

My Personal Need for Support

In the discussions following my presentations, some people have picked up the apparent inconsistency in my need for someone close, to touch me, and to become deeply involved in my life, and my feeling of growing separation and aloneness. This is another of the emotional paradoxes I have lived with these long months. I believe in the need for personal involvement and I believe in its power. But people can get only so far into your life. The limits are set by both persons involved.

Even though I am aware of my separation from those whom I love the most, the support they offer me is valid. And I must have this in order to survive.

I realize I am closing people out of my life. I am closing Gordon out of my life. It's just the way dying is operating in my life. If there were some other way for me to resolve my final separation, I would do it.

This need for support is closely related to my desire to control my own life and destiny. One of the most helpful ways people can support me is by allowing me to maintain control. When I see that I am losing control by people determining what's best for me and suggesting how I'm going to respond, my defense mechanism is to withdraw — to keep people out of my life. This I have done to Gordon when I can't cope with the threat of losing control. But still I need him — the support he offers — and the ability to maintain the control which only he can give me.

To offer support in a short-term crisis and over an extended period of time creates two different needs for me and for those around me.

When no one thought I would live beyond a few months, it was relatively easy to provide the support I needed. And I must admit that need was basically an ego need. I remember one girl who came to me in a meeting and said, "I've always wanted to tell you, but tonight I will say it for sure because of the way things are. I think you are a wonderful person."

That helped take away some of the bitterness I was experiencing — far more than the "jolly cards" I received. But it was good for her as well. We all grow when we give and receive "strokes."

Now, to keep that support going over an extended period of time is difficult, if not impossible. While I crave that, I'm not sure it is best for me, because continually feeding my ego becomes a game and makes me think I am more than the person I am.

So the most difficult problem is for the family to remain consistent in their support, for, on the one hand, I want to be treated as I always have been so as not to be reminded of my terminal illness. I want my family and friends to be themselves. On the other hand, I find myself constantly manipulating those closest to me to gain the emotional support I want.

I often feel that the only way I can get the support I need is to become dependent. But I can't take that step — at least not yet. Gordon tells me I must learn to be "independently dependent." That's pretty impossible. I can hardly stand to think of becoming dependent, so I say and do things I shouldn't to show people I will remain independent. I'm very angry because things haven't worked as I planned them. When that anger is evident, it is almost impossible for my family and friends to give me support.

The longer I live and the healthier I look, the more difficult it is to offer support. Even Gordon says in response to "How's JoAnn doing?" — "She's doing whatever she puts her mind to." And I suppose that's true but it comes out of sheer guts, not because I feel like it. It takes all the energy I can muster just to cope with the problems of our foster children. Others who are less strong and more dependent get more attention and the kind of support I want. But I can never be happy being that way. Since I can't have my cake and eat it too, prolonged illness continues to make me ambivalent, and this has created part of the reason for my intense emotional highs and lows.

One of the most supportive feelings I have experienced is acceptance of the kind of person I now am. I was once attractive. Now at age forty-nine I am bloated and I've lost my hair; my anger, depression, and hostility are hard to take. My personality has been altered many times.

It's very hard to believe that my husband, a man in the prime of his life, still loves a woman as ugly as all that.

To have the assurance of his acceptance and that of the rest of the family, our foster children, and my friends, is the kind of help I really need.

Emotionally and spiritually, we have a deep relationship with a dozen friends. They are with us on a gut level day or night, sunshine or rain, whether I'm a bitch or not. And that's a miracle for which I can never thank God enough.

The one really wonderful thing that has come to me during my suffering is in relationships. There have been no ecstatic visitations of heavenly creatures — the only angel who visited me was the girl in white who came from the nursing station to give me my shot. Our relationships have been most meaningful in our religious community. In those moments I know I'm not alone. Jesus is really with me — in the flesh of those who care and who stay by me no matter what.

Those Cards and Letters

I have received a number of letters and cards from people who heard or read of my illness and have wanted to offer their support. I have divided them between the "goodies" and the "baddies." The bad ones are unreal. Many of them had remedies including suggestions for secret treatments in Mexico, a variety of new underground drugs and health diets, which, by the way, all include carrot juice — that seems to be a "biggy" in helping to cure cancer. Some of them reminded me that "if you have faith, you will be cured." Some of the letters were four or five pages long!

These letters all made me feel quite sad because I consider myself a Christian operating the best way I can under the circumstances. The new cures imply my choice of medical care is wrong even though I have accepted the fact that there is no cure for cancer and, as a result, know I am going to die of that disease, barring some unforeseen and unexpected miracle. And it is hard to take correspondence from fellow Christians implying my experience with Christ isn't real or I would be healed.

I would say I was almost harassed by proponents of the "anti-cancer" drug Laetrile, a chemical extracted from the kernels of apricot pits. They are evangelists in promoting its use as a treatment or preventive of cancer. I was even invited to a rally in Rochester, Minnesota, attended by over eight hundred sympathizers, on March 26, 1974. Although its effectiveness is unproven by the medical establishment, including cancer specialists, the Food and Drug Administration, and the American Cancer Society, its proponents will help you find the right doctor and will help doctors get access to Laetrile.

The professor of a graduate student friend of mine at the University of Minnesota was so impressed by the fact that people took time to write such long letters to someone they hadn't even met, that he asked the student to make a study of them and she fulfilled an academic requirement with her report.

There's another group of people — also church-type and maybe even Christian — who send me cards and letters telling me to look up, get well, and with other similar simplistic messages. I'm not going to

118

get well, and the flowers aren't blooming, nor the sun shining — most of the time! I'm having a hard time coping with just getting through the day with my drugs and trying to be halfway civil to people and make some contribution to our foster children and be a decent wife. Those cards and letters just don't speak to where I am. Because they add to my depression, they are of more harm than they are of help.

Better than the cards advising me to "look up," "have faith," and "be of good cheer" are the ones which simply state a fact. Of course, who sends the card is important, too, and whether or not the message is consistent with the sender. A little Peanuts character card that said, "Happiness is being home," was just about perfect because it came from a close friend who also is a cancer patient.

It's easier to send messages about the power of prayer and keeping a stiff upper lip than it is for most people to cope with the facts — how long will it be? how do you really feel?

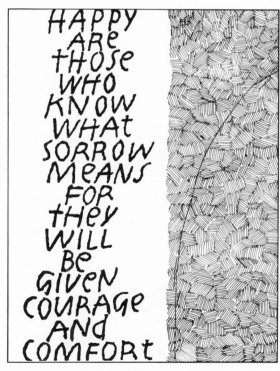

"Better than the cards advising me to 'look up,' 'have faith,' and 'be of good cheer' are the ones that simply state a fact."

HAPPY ARE THOSE WHO KNOW WHAT SORROW MEANS FOR THEY WILL BE GIVEN COURAGE AND COMFORT

By Courtesy of: Conception Abbey Press
Conception, Missouri
CA 1088

Spiritual Support

Someone asked me if I would welcome spiritual support from my nurses. I said, "Yes, but define what you mean by 'spiritual.' " I have had little girl nurses think they gave me that kind of support when they prayed in my ear and said nice things which were most inappropriate for the kind of person I am.

But if a nurse came in, or anyone for that matter, and wanted to discuss my faith with me, I would welcome that, provided it were a fair exchange; that is, provided she has something to offer me and she is willing to accept me in return. But no easy answers, please. As a matter of fact never *any* answer, like "a miracle could happen" or "you're going to get well." That's religiosity — not spirituality.

A humanist could offer me more support than that if he was a real humanist and if he was sincere and open.

To me, the most important aspect of spiritual support is the honest encounter I have when people share with me their feelings about life and death. Spiritual support is offered by those who help me use the faith I possess to confront the reality of my situation or who act out their own faith on my behalf without insisting that I believe as they do. Religiosity is thrusting their beliefs on me.

Spiritual support has come to me in many ways. Some of it has not even been verbalized. But acts on my behalf from people of all faiths have sustained me in a way I can't describe adequately.

"All six of my kids got up early this morning and prayed for you," John told me the morning of the liver biopsy. The vision of those children who believed in the efficacy of prayer moved me deeply and gave me renewed strength. Another Catholic friend wrote to her priest brother in Korea, who said a special mass for me and then wrote to me. That same friend fasted during Lent as a spiritual gift, and she gave me a symbol of the Holy Spirit that I cherish. She has faithfully prayed for me, offered herself on my behalf to God, and lighted candles as symbols of her prayers for my courage to endure.

My own religious community assures me of their spiritual support every time we meet — embracing and touching me to assure me I am still here, and they are with me.

One of the most beautiful and supportive experiences Agora provided for me was on February 25, 1973, three days before I was released from the hospital. One of Gail's unfinished pieces of business she wanted to complete while I was still alive was to make her public confession of faith and her baptism.

She talked with her dad often about this and when he was convinced her motives were real and not just a desire to please her mother, the two of them met with the Agora Community and decided to have a commitment service in my hospital room. And if I lived, then I could witness her public baptism.

Several adults, members of the family, including our foster children, and her personal friends crowded into my room. Following some informal singing, a specially prepared litany, Scripture, and sharing, Gail was asked if she believed in Christ as her Savior and if she intended to be baptized by immersion at the earliest convenient date. She responded by saying, "Yes." We then observed the Lord's Supper, which I led, using elements made by members of Agora as their gifts to this meaningful experience.

"It was really neat," Gail recorded in her diary. Her commitment was made public on a Friday evening, March 16, 1973, when I was in attendance.

One of my strongest personal needs is for a priest. Maybe that sounds funny from a Protestant, and a Baptist, at that. But when I was sure I was going to die, my friend John Sundquist heard my confession and said, "Sister, in the name of Jesus Christ I assure you your sins are forgiven." That gave me a real sense of well-being and peace.

A few weeks later he moved out of the area and my friend Alice assumed that role. I have talked with her many times and confessed all my inner fears and feelings. My great fear is that she won't be there when the final hour comes.

The Christian needs that support. If one's pastor has fulfilled the role of shepherd and priest during one's life, he can do so at death. But that role can be filled by anyone sensitive to the needs of the dying person and on the same spiritual and theological wave length. What a fantastic ministry for lay people seeking more meaning for their own Christian experience!

Family Support

The family of a dying patient offers the greatest support when the members are as open and honest in their communications as they can be. Don't hide things from the dying person or you set up real blocks in communication. Relate to them as if they are physically healthy but don't be afraid to talk about death. Tell them how much they mean to you and don't be afraid to grieve.

Sometimes such an attempt may mean we will be emotionally hurt and we'll suffer pain, but that is part of caring.

I have sometimes felt my family has not supported me as much as they could have. But I have often reconstructed my reaction to my mother's death and from it have found insight into how my own growing family reacts to the death of a parent.

I was living in Seattle, pregnant with Brian, when my father called and suggested I should come home. My mother was angered by that although he and my sister had checked with a physician in North Platte, Nebraska, where they were, and discovered that I was in the best time of pregnancy for safety in traveling. Mother was angry because pregnancy for me had come hard, and she didn't want anything to happen to me or the baby.

When my mother died shortly after I arrived, I did not express the grief or sorrow in the same way that my family did. But I have felt deep grief since that time. I have mourned for my mother during these long years — especially on the important occasions in the life of our family when I really wished she could have been here to share our joy.

But my baby was coming. And I was so happy for that long-awaited event that it seemed to displace the grief I would have otherwise experienced.

Our three children, in a similar way, are excited about life, which is opening for them as they mature into young adults. Life work, choice of college, dating, the importance of their peer group — all tend to displace the reality of our impending separation.

"They should pay more attention to me," I think. But they don't. Intellectually I can identify with where they are, for I was where they are when my mother died — with the possible exception of Gail, who is entering her last two years of high school. Her life is still wrapped up in the home and her parents. She will have the toughest time of all, for her life experiences are limited in comparison with her older brother and sister.

Gordon has felt a strong need for us to have more time alone during my illness. He feels squeezed out from time he wants alone with me. I have not disagreed with this, but I have not responded readily to his suggestions to go out alone or even to make a trip without someone else.

There were two notable exceptions. And they fit into our general philosophy of doing what we want to do when we want.

In the winter of 1973, Gordon convinced me to go to Las Vegas for three days. We had never been there and never really were turned on by what that city had to offer. But we enjoy life, entertainment, and good food. Since these "goodies" were all centered on the renowned "strip," we wouldn't need to travel or walk a lot, which was one of the factors which kept us from other traveling experiences during my illness. We could sleep when we wanted to, eat when the spirit moved, and just plain be together away from pressures of our extended family and others.

That was a great experience. We enjoyed just being with each other.

In the spring of 1974, Gordon convinced me a second time to get away on our own. I finally gave in. It was a Thursday night, and by the following afternoon we had checked into a Minneapolis hotel for a "pampered-in-pink" package weekend.

I was very tired and slept most of the time while Gordon worked on the manuscript for this book. But we had time to talk out some very important things and were very happy we made that effort.

Other times when we tried to go out alone it turned out to be a disaster — primarily because I was emotionally down and very hostile.

So most of the time we arranged our social life in the presence of others, and my temperament would be inhibited by them.

This hurt Gordon, but he seemed to accept the reality of this new style of life. My own needs were met better by a group of people. And I preferred occasions that gave me a chance to talk about my fears, uncertainty, apprehension, and feelings. So I became turned off by movies and the theater, which had been such an important part of our life in earlier years.

I have stated that people need people. But another of the great needs a human has is the need to be needed. I believe that is more real in the dying person than in anyone else.

Our home has offered that kind of support to me. Most of the time I have felt really needed by our foster children. In my depression I have often doubted this, but in my better moments I know this is true.

Several of our foster children have made this clear to me many different times. Two are now married. One of them saw her mother die of cancer, and one night in our family group meeting she said, "Since I was nine years old, I have been looking for a woman who could offer me what I needed from a mother. I have found that person in JoAnn. I know she can't be my mother — and I wouldn't take her away from Paula and Gail. But she's the only one I've been able to relate to on a gut level. Now I must find someone else. Will I always have to find a new person to give me what I need?"

My family has reacted to my periods of remission by entering a denial stage of sorts; that is, they knew I wasn't going to die that day or even that week. But I still want them to show their care like they did when they thought I would be gone soon. I want them to say every day, "You know, Mother, I love you and need you." And then kiss me. Then I'd know their need for me is real.

Hope

The answer to the terminally ill patients' great emotional needs is coming both from the health care professionals and from the patients themselves.

For example, in the Veterans Administration Hospital of Palo Alto, California, group discussions between staff and terminally ill patients were begun in June of 1972 to meet the psychosocial needs of patients and to help all participants learn more about death and dying. The patients have learned openness and offered their support to each other as together they confront questions relative to their family, their pain, and their relationship to God.

Staff members follow up the meetings with individual counseling based on their personal relationships with the patient.

Hope as a support mechanism for the terminal patient was the motivation for a movement that began in Burlington, Iowa, in January of 1974 and almost overnight swept the nation. M.T.C., or Make Today Count, is the brainchild of a forty-two-year old newsman, Orville Kelley, terminally ill with cancer, who organized a chapter in his home to help cancer victims get over the depression, impatience, and lonely feelings so familiar to all who share this disease. Kelley found it impossible to live with his fits of depression and decided there must be a better way than self-pity and anger.

His monthly meetings are "to share experiences that foster growth and understanding," and the "springboard is hope."

Through meetings of cancer victims and their families, thousands of people have learned to live in the present — now — getting the most out of each minute of the day.

M.T.C. chapters have sprung up "like dandelions" both in the United States and Europe. And the estimated 265,000 people who die of cancer in 1974 and the 1,300,000 who each year will discover they have it have found a new source of hope — in sharing their problems and in supporting each other.

M.T.C. puts out a regular newsletter which offers help to cancer victims through the personal stories of members and their expressions of their feelings through poetry and other writings.

The opportunity for a church or an organization within the church to give leadership in organizing a local chapter is a tremendous opportunity for mission in any community. Many cancer victims, like me, would welcome the opportunity to participate but fail to have the strength or time to give the leadership to form such a group.

M.T.C. illustrates the need for hope and the hope which we cancer victims can give each other in moments of depression and despair.

It is this sense of hope which offers me the greatest support to cope with life as I now experience it. This is not so much the hope I wrote of earlier, which has to do with my ultimate destiny. But it is hope for the more immediate future — a sort of an existential hope, if that isn't redundant.

I had hoped to see my fifteen-year-old reach her sixteenth birthday. And now I hope to see her seventeenth. I had hoped to live long enough to see Paula graduate from high school. Now I hope to see her complete her second year of college.

I hope to see some real changes in the lives of the teenagers in our house.

I hoped to see my first two foster daughters married.

I hope to live long enough to see my second "foster" grandchild.

Now I hope to have strength enough to meet my next speaking engagement.

And that's not a superficial hope.

And with this hope for more life is the hope that I will remain consistently a God-person in the midst of pain and under the influence of medication, so that I can be true to my friends, family, and my faith — to the end.

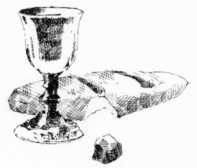

On an April Sunday, in 1974, members of the Agora Community were seated in a circle with the elements of the Lord's Supper on a table in the center. We were each asked to come up, speak or pray, take the elements, and return to our seat.

When my turn came, I moved to the table and said, "I pray for another year of life." I was weeping so much I could hardly take the elements — and there were others around that circle who could not hide their emotions either.

When hope for another day — another experience — another relationship is gone, then my motivation for living will die, too.

And the death of JoAnn Smith will be imminent.

125

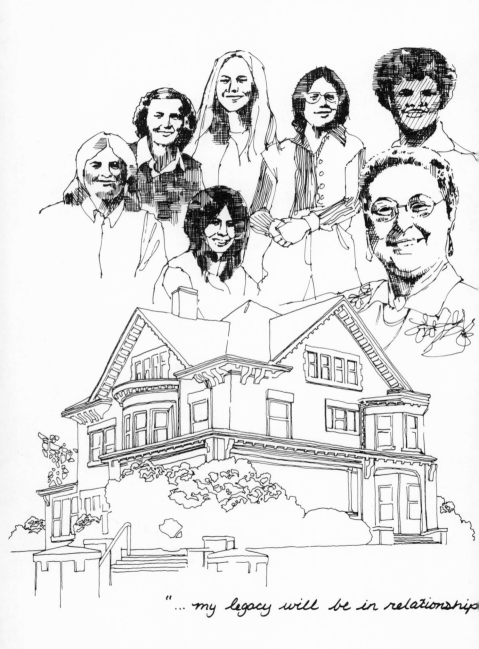

"... my legacy will be in relationship"

Mother is getting around a little bit more now. She has her good days and bad ones. There was one day though that I'll never forget. She seemed very sick so Paula and I stayed home from school. Brian came over that afternoon. Mother decided that we should take care of her things and relinquish them to their new owners. This would be hard for her, but she did it in the most dignified way, and with great respect. That was a day I really felt close to her. She brought me into her bedroom and asked me if there was a certain ring that I would like. Mother held three rings that I liked, but there was one I'd always especially admired. I told her tearfully because I didn't exactly feel right saying I wanted it. She detected this and said, "This was mine once but now it is yours. When you wear it, remember me and how much I love you and always will." I just gave her a great big kiss and hug to show her I understood and felt the same way without saying it. I had a hard time with words then.

Then I left and let somebody else go in. It was their turn to have a private time with her. The rest of the day she divided her other things, but they will never be as important as the ring she gave to me.

So Gail described the way I decided to begin my preparation for death. It was after my return from the hospital in February of 1973, and I felt time was short. I had some very close moments with my family and friends. Brian and Paula were now independent, but I was concerned about Gail and the turbulent teenage years still uncompleted. But she assured me, "You needn't worry — I'll cause no problem for Dad."

My personal items were distributed to my children, and all dishes, antiques — anything of sentimental value — were marked; if I had a preference for who should get them, I said so.

Gordon and I took inventory of our assets and discussed final disposition of property jointly held. In one way, perhaps, I was fortunate in having time to think things through and to get whatever legal advice we needed.

In our case we had wills drawn up several years ago. Our attorney advised us to transfer all property into single ownership, in Gordon's name, making probate of my will unnecessary since there would then be no estate.

This was done.

I have thought a great deal about the legacy I offer those whom I love and realize it's not in things, as meaningful and as sentimental as some of those may be. I hope my legacy will be in relationships. My highest ambition has always been to make a difference in people's lives. To that end I have cultivated deep personal relationships, which have enriched my life — and, I hope, theirs.

Out of her Indian tradition, Elizabeth Walters Higgins sent me this tribal song:

> **See the morning**
> **See the mysterious mountain**
> **Something marvelous and sacred**
> **though it happens every day**
> **Dawn the child of God and Darkness.**
> **All things moving**
> **New day coming**
> **Life renewing.**

To this poem she added her personal note, affirming the legacy I pray will be mine:

> **Life is renewed in so many ways.**
> **I think many lives are going to be**
> **renewed through yours.**

I have expressed my deep appreciation to several people who have always accepted me just as I am — with my strong opinions and in times of great happiness and deep sadness. Their impact on me, particularly in the long months of my illness, can never be measured. And, hopefully, I will leave them with memories and experiences that have made them better people because we have known each other and have fulfilled one of the greatest of human desires — that of needing each other.

One of these friends responded to my discouragement and loss of hope in the many months of my illness and my questioning of its meaning by saying, with tears in her eyes, "But I need you."

And another, a friend from college days, wrote after I had spoken in her church, "Your words made me realize anew what a precious thing is life, and how unique is the role of each one of us. Also they remind me again of the perspective with which a true Christian can view each day's events and responsibilities."

But the most meaningful legacy is the relationship I have enjoyed with the young people in our home. Many were frustrating. Many disappointing. But there were a few that made it all worthwhile.

For example, on Mother's Day, 1974, I received this letter from Linda and her husband, Doug. Gordon performed their wedding shortly after she left our home to establish an independent life.

I hope that this is a very happy Mother's Day for you. You deserve the very best because without you my life would probably be rotten. You've taught me love, patience, and understanding, and most of all when to say no. You've helped me graduate from high school and to fall in love with the most wonderful man in the world. I think that the greatest thing that you did for me was helping me fulfill my wedding dream.

Thank you, JoAnn, for everything else. When we have our first little girl, we're going to name her JoAnn in hopes that she will be as wise and wonderful as you!

Because I believe relationships are my only real legacy, I have arranged to have memorial funds established: (1) to remind people of what they have meant to me, and (2) to encourage others to discover how much they need another human being.

One fund would be established with the Agora Community to be used to encourage the young people of our religious community — through scholarships for camp, college, or to provide any other experience that would help them grow into mature Christians.

The other would go to the Baptist Hospital Fund, Inc., of St. Paul, which sponsors Mounds-Midway School of Nursing, where the door was opened for me to begin my new vocation interpreting my feelings about death. The Baptist Hospital Fund also sponsors Midway Hospital, and Gordon and I both owe a deep debt of gratitude for the compassionate care I received there and for the thoughtful concern of its staff headed by L. M. Conley, the executive director. Through my care at Midway, I learned the value of human relationships in confronting the deepest of human crises.

The memorial service presented some difficulty for us as I admit to several hang-ups in my theological position with respect to the body and its disposition.

On the one hand, I recognize the Christian position that the real JoAnn is not the disease-ridden body I have, but it's that spirit or personality that makes me who I am.

129

On the other hand, my body is the visible me. It has been described by the apostle Paul as "a temple of the Holy Spirit" and we are admonished to treat it with sacred respect and care (I Corinthians 6:19-20).

I do not regard my body as nothing — but as something of such great importance that I want it treated with respect and dignity.

The finality of death and the end of all human relationships are affirmed when one sees a lifeless corpse in a coffin. I will never forget that impression after seeing both my parents in death. And I want my family to experience that, so there is never a question about the finality of my death.

The funeral experience also offers a therapeutic opportunity for grief to be expressed. I believe that is healthy, leaving fewer emotional scars than if I suddenly am absent and there is nobody over which to express grief. As Charlie Brown would say, that's "good grief."

For these reasons, some pastors, theologians, and psychologists are once again promoting the open-casket "visitation" and the presence of the body in a traditional funeral service. I heard a psychologist say once that when he dies he would like to have his body dressed in a red Chinese mandarin costume, carried by friends, lifted above mourners, Eastern style, through the streets. Bells would be clanging and friends shouting, "He's gone to be with God."

But Gordon and I have long felt that the American way of death has become obscene. There is too much spent on putting the body to rest that could be used to improve the quality of life for the living. And the responsibility is not totally that of the funeral industry, for expensive funerals are often demanded by relatives and loved ones who, in bereavement, want to show their love through lavishness.

One mortuary quotes Gladstone in its brochure advertising its services: "Show me the manner in which a nation cares for its dead, and I will measure with exactness the tender mercies of its people, their respect for the laws of the land, and their loyalty to high ideals."

The multibillion dollar funeral business of the United States hardly proves this.

There are many voices raised pleading for us to restore the human values of the past. Well, in the pre-Civil War days a "good Christian burial" cost about twenty-five dollars. Now the expectations of one's family and friends have raised that to well over one thousand dollars.

And with our increased spending to show respect for the dead, the values cited by Gladstone seem to be more obscure. The traditional funeral perpetuates the materialism which surrounds the idolatry of the body. This idolatry has its litany and sacred music in the advertising

130

which saturates the media. It's not the person that is of value but how that person dresses, how he looks, and the cars he drives. Bodies represent employment statistics, the ability to produce and consume.

Persons feel!

And the idolatry comes when we make the image of people as producers and consumers our god and worship it with the spending of our time and our money.

Gordon and I both identify strongly with John Carmody's account of his father's funeral:

> The memory of my father's funeral is also fraught with anger. I found the religious establishment even more offensive than the medical. The failure of Christian leaders to end or transform the ancient custom of "waking" the dead is incomprehensible. I found my father's two-day wake a shocking perversity, and largely an exercise in evasion. The wake is a psychological phenomenon and a religious abomination. It is another structured superficiality. One has to be strong indeed if one is to transform it from a morbid get-together into anything reverent of mystery. Neither real grief nor Easter faith is welcome at a wake . . . .[1]

My memorial service will seek to affirm the Christian posture in the style of our religious community.

The first thing we did was to take out a lifetime membership of ten dollars per person with the Minnesota Memorial Society, which provides burial service ranging in price from $250 to $385. There are 120 member societies throughout the United States and Canada. Wherever they are located, there are cooperating mortuaries, which, by the way, often do not enjoy the cooperation or well wishes of their professional peers.

If my body were not so diseased and marred, I would have bequeathed it and my organs to the University of Minnesota, as Gordon has done.

At my death, the immediate family will gather for interment as soon as possible at a cemetery sponsored by the Minnesota Memorial Society. My death will provide the occasion for viewing my lifeless body and will offer an outlet for expressions of grief.

The memorial service will be held a week or ten days later, in the evening, for the convenience of those who want to join in celebration for my life.

---

[1] John Carmody, "A Death, a Radicalization," *The Christian Century* (vol. 91, no. 23), June 12-19, 1974, p. 640.

The service will be in three parts:
1. The affirmation of the religious community in life and death.
2. The acknowledgment of the reality of death.
3. The celebration of life's meaning.

Traditional and contemporary music will be played by an organist, a guitarist, and a Dixieland band. The latter group also will play at a reception where, I hope, there will be dancing and lots of love for life expressed through good conversation, eating, and drinking together.

There will be multimedia presentations with slides and tapes of appropriate music. Scripture, prayer, and litany will be led by women who have been close to me.

And there will be open sharing of what this experience has meant to members of our family, our foster children, my physician, and my friends — Some will share with the whole group and others on a one-to-one basis with those seated next to them — in the style of Agora worship.

Poetry and prose which I have chosen to represent my feelings about death — some as traditional as Scripture and others as contemporary as Dag Hammarskjöld — will be projected through the use of slides.

And the sanctuary will be decorated with banners.

The most prominent will be the largest. It will be in the center of the sanctuary chancel. It will affirm the reality of the resurrection in new relationships and situations where Christ again reveals himself as he did on the road to Emmaus.

It will symbolize what I feel my death experience has meant for me. And the hope for those who remain.

For it is my banner. I made it for Gail's baptism.

It is deep blue with a gold sun rising in the background.

And in the foreground are the words:

HERE COMES THE SUN.

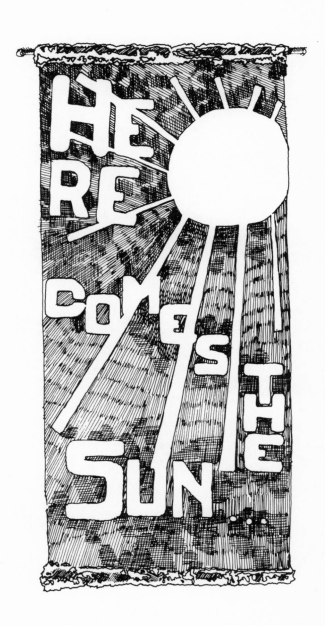

Epilogue

Gordon Smith

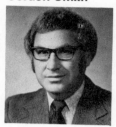

JoAnn was admitted to the University Hospitals at the University of Minnesota, in Minneapolis, on Friday, October 14, 1974. She was transferred from Midway Hospital to determine if the neurologist there could find an alternative to medication for the pain that had become almost intolerable.

During her ten days there, her condition deteriorated, and when she became jaundiced, tests were given to determine if her condition was related to the progress of her disease.

I called the doctor at 9:30 A.M., October 25, to inquire about test results after efforts the previous day had failed to get this information from the hospital's nursing staff.

I learned later that she had vomited blood during the night.

I am still haunted by the thought of that scene and cannot believe she did not ask for me. After our ordeal of twenty-one months, I certainly could have given another nine hours of support when it was needed most. But I was never officially informed of her critical condition by those responsible for her care.

Because the doctor was not alarmed, I responded similarly and asked if she could be transferred back to Midway. He agreed to make the necessary arrangements immediately.

A nurse friend who cared for JoAnn at Midway and who had participated as a graduate student in several sessions which JoAnn led on death and dying, made two quick calls to me, shortly after 10:00 A.M., insisting that I get to the hospital as soon as possible. In her opinion JoAnn was in no condition to be moved.

She had agreed to keep close track of JoAnn's progress while in University Hospitals since it was impossible for me to see her as often as I did when she was a patient at Midway. She had forced herself into the intensive care unit that morning against the regulations of the hospital. "You don't understand how critical her condition is," she told me. She had been able to communicate with JoAnn and learned that I had not been there since she began hemorrhaging. She couldn't believe that and called me to confirm what JoAnn had said.

When I arrived at 11:15 A.M., I found her to be very uncomfortable,

137

with I.V.'s and blood transfusions being administered. "We can't stop the internal bleeding without surgery," the resident told me.

When I acted astonished, he added, "That would be heroics uncalled for in this situation." I then asked to have all equipment removed, assuring him that JoAnn and I had often talked about this kind of situation and we were prepared to face the consequences.

JoAnn was still restless so I suggested to the nurse that medication be administered to make her comfortable.

Our friend called Brian, Paula, Gail, and Gladys. Brian was soon at his mother's bedside, and with him holding one hand, me the other, and with Gladys's arms around the two of us, we watched her die. Her love and professional skill helped us through those last three hours as she interpreted the signs of approaching death.

When it appeared that JoAnn had lost all awareness, I whispered to Brian, "I think she's taken her last conscious breath — she's taken her leap of faith."

The fear of death she articulated on so many occasions was not evident.

Neither was there a denial of faith. She had often expressed concern that because of her suffering and pain — and the alteration of her personality — she might come to the end cursing God and blaming others. Her fear was groundless.

In the last two months of her life JoAnn experienced a dramatic change in her outlook and in her personality. Her denial of death was not as obvious as in the compulsiveness she evidenced the preceding months. The anger, resentment, loneliness, anxiety, fear — about which she wrote — all gave way to a more loving nature, an attitude of reconciliation, and a spirit of acceptance.

In her life there was a restlessness — to discover — to achieve — to find purpose — to be creative. But there was an inner peace which grounded her in her restlessness.

And in her last hours the same restless spirit was present. There was the desire to control what was happening to her. When she wanted her hand held, she offered it. When she wanted it free, she pulled it away.

But when she could no longer fight for the life she loved so much, she became still.

She died quietly.

Her facial expression was that of peace.

And we learned what many tried to tell us through the long months of her illness.

We die the way we live.

JoAnn died at 1:30 P.M. Friday, October 25, 1974 . . . .

138

. . . to be continued.